Pain, the Opioid Epidemic, & Depression

Pain, the Opioid Epidemic, & Depression

Edited by
JEFFREY F. SCHERRER &
JANE C. BALLANTYNE

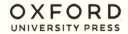

OXFORD
UNIVERSITY PRESS

Oxford University Press is a department of the University of Oxford.
It furthers the University's objective of excellence in research, scholarship,
and education by publishing worldwide. Oxford is a registered trade mark of
Oxford University Press in the UK and in certain other countries.

Published in the United States of America by Oxford University Press
198 Madison Avenue, New York, NY 10016, United States of America.

© Oxford University Press 2024

All rights reserved. No part of this publication may be reproduced, stored in
a retrieval system, or transmitted, in any form or by any means, without the
prior permission in writing of Oxford University Press, or as expressly permitted
by law, by license or under terms agreed with the appropriate reprographics
rights organization. Inquiries concerning reproduction outside the scope of the
above should be sent to the Rights Department, Oxford University Press, at the
address above.

You must not circulate this work in any other form
and you must impose this same condition on any acquirer

Library of Congress Cataloging-in-Publication Data
Names: Scherrer, Jeffrey F., editor. | Ballantyne, Jane, 1948– editor.
Title: Pain, the opioid epidemic, & depression / Jeffrey F. Scherrer, editor;
Jane C. Ballantyne, co-editor.
Description: New York, NY : Oxford University Press, [2024] |
Includes bibliographical references and index.
Identifiers: LCCN 2024006436 (print) | LCCN 2024006437 (ebook) |
ISBN 9780197675229 (hardback) | ISBN 9780197675243 (epub) | ISBN 9780197675250
Subjects: MESH: Chronic Pain—drug therapy | Opioid Epidemic |
Pain Management | Depression—drug therapy | Analgesics,
Opioid—adverse effects | Opioid-Related Disorders | United States
Classification: LCC RC568.O45 (print) | LCC RC568.O45 (ebook) |
NLM WL 704.6 | DDC 362.29/3—dc23/eng/20240401
LC record available at https://lccn.loc.gov/2024006436
LC ebook record available at https://lccn.loc.gov/2024006437

DOI: 10.1093/9780197675250.001.0001

Printed by Integrated Books International, United States of America

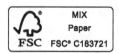

To my wife, Leslie Scherrer, and my beautiful children, Hannah, Emma, and Zachary; your love and support make it all possible. Sincere appreciation to collaborators and colleagues who have contributed to this book.

—Jeffrey F. Scherrer

To all those people who have encouraged me to keep up the fight for better pain management.

—Jane C. Ballantyne

Contents

Acknowledgments	xi
List of Abbreviations and Acronyms	xiii
List of Contributors	xv

1. Overview and Purpose
Jeffrey F. Scherrer and Jane C. Ballantyne

1.1	Introduction	1
1.2	Chapter Overview	2
1.3	Key Concepts to Assist Readers	5
1.4	Overview of the Non-Cancer Pain, Opioid Epidemic, and Depression Tripartite	7
1.5	Clinical and Public Health Relevance	10

1

2. Neurophysiology of Pain, Depression, and Exogenous Opioids
Geoffrey Panjeton and Hess Amir Panjeton

2.1	Introduction	13
2.2	Neurophysiological Mechanisms Underlying Comorbid Pain and Depression	13
2.3	Common Underlying Physiology	14
2.4	The Role of Opioid Medications on the Link Between Pain and Depression	16
2.5	Hedonic Capacity Related to Chronic Opioid Use	18
2.6	Conclusion	19

13

3. Looking Beyond Tissue Damage: Pain as a Homeostatic Emotion
Mark D. Sullivan

3.1	Introduction	21
3.2	Alternative View: Pain as Interoceptive Homeostatic Emotion	22
3.3	Colin Klein's Imperative Theory of Pain	24
3.4	Pain in the Brain: From Pain Matrix to Salience Network	25
3.5	The Relation of Pain to Hurt and Suffering	28
3.6	Pain, Anxiety, and Depression as Homeostatic Emotions	29
3.7	Opioids, Pain, and Depression	32
3.8	Conclusion	33

21

viii CONTENTS

4. Prescription Opioid Use and Risk of Depression and
Worsening Mental Health 37
Jeffrey F. Scherrer and Joanne Salas
  4.1 Overview 37
  4.2 Measuring Non-Cancer Pain 38
  4.3 Defining Long-Term Opioid Therapy 39
  4.4 Considerations for Standardizing Dosage 40
  4.5 Pain as a Key Confounding Factor 40
  4.6 Propensity Scores and Inverse Probability of Treatment
Weighting 42
  4.7 Summary of Evidence from Existing Cross-Sectional Studies 44
  4.8 Results from Existing Retrospective Cohort Studies:
Risks for New-Onset Depression 45
  4.9 Evidence from Retrospective Cohort Studies: LTOT and
Risk for Depression 48
  4.10 Results from Prospective Cohort Studies 49
  4.11 Escalating Dose and Frequency of Use May Explain
Risk for New-Onset Depression 51
  4.12 Is Depression a Side Effect or Consequence of Long-Term
Opioid Use? 53
  4.13 Does Opioid Use Lead Specifically to Major Depressive
Episodes or to Psychopathology in General? 53
  4.14 Does Long-Term Prescription Opioid Use Cause Depression? 54
  4.15 Potential Biological Mechanisms 55
  4.16 Psychosocial Mechanisms 56
  4.17 Public Health and Clinical Relevance 57
  4.18 Conclusion 57

5. Depression and Pain: Bidirectional Relationship and
Changes with Psychological Treatment 62
Lisa R. Miller-Matero
  5.1 Introduction 62
  5.2 Psychological Treatments for Co-Occurring Chronic
Pain and Depression 63
  5.3 Psychological Interventions to Reduce Prescription
Opioid Use Among Individuals with Chronic Pain 67
  5.4 Challenges in Managing Comorbid Pain, Depression, and
Opioid Use and Potential Solutions 68
  5.5 Conclusion 71

6. Other Psychiatric Disorders, Psychosocial Factors, Sleep, and
Pain 80
Matthew J. Bair and Ashli A. Owen-Smith
  6.1 Introduction 80
  6.2 Chronic Pain and Anxiety 81

CONTENTS   ix

6.3	Chronic Pain and Posttraumatic Stress Disorder	88
6.4	Chronic Pain and Bipolar Disorder	93
6.5	Pain and Schizophrenia	97
6.6	Research Gaps and Future Directions for the Study of Comorbid Chronic Pain and Psychiatric Disorders	102
6.7	Conclusion	103

7. The Impact of Social and Structural Determinants on Depression, Prescription Opioid Use, Opioid Misuse, and Opioid Use Disorder   117

Fred Rottnek and Jennifer K. Bello-Kottenstette

7.1	Introduction	117
7.2	Impact of Economic Stability	118
7.3	Impact of Education Access and Quality	121
7.4	Impact of Healthcare Access and Quality	123
7.5	Impact of Neighborhood and Built Environment	125
7.6	Impact of Social and Community Context and Connectedness	127
7.7	Conclusion	129

8. Opioid Taper and Complex Prescription Opioid Dependence: The Role of Depression   138

Travis I. Lovejoy and Belle Zaccari

8.1	Introduction	138
8.2	Defining Opioid Dependence	139
8.3	Pain and Endogenous Opioid Systems	140
8.4	Opponent Processes	140
8.5	Allostasis	141
8.6	Depression in the Context of Opioid Use and Opioid Taper	142
8.7	Treatment in Interdisciplinary Pain Programs During Opioid Taper	142
8.8	Future Research Directions	143
8.9	Conclusion	145

9. Potential Role for Buprenorphine in the Management of Comorbid Depression Among People with Chronic Pain and Long-Term Opioid Therapy Dependence   148

Ajay Manhapra, Robert Rosenheck, and William C. Becker

9.1	Introduction	148
9.2	History of Therapeutic Use of Buprenorphine to Treat Depression	149
9.3	Buprenorphine Basic Pharmacology	152
9.4	Low-Dose Buprenorphine in Treatment-Refractory Depression Among Opioid-Naïve Individuals	153
9.5	Buprenorphine in Treatment of Depression Comorbid with Opioid Use Disorder	154

X CONTENTS

9.6 Buprenorphine in Treatment of Depression Comorbid
with Chronic Pain and Long-Term Opioid Therapy 155
9.7 How Long-Term Opioid Use for Pain Can Lead to More
Pain and Depression 157
9.8 Buprenorphine Use in LTOT Dependence-Induced
OICP and Associated Depression 158
9.9 Conclusion 160

10. Future Directions in Pain Management: Implications for
Depression and Mental Health 165
Jane C. Ballantyne, Mark D. Sullivan, and Jeffrey F. Scherrer
10.1 Research to Determine If Treating Depression and Other
Psychiatric Disorders to Remission Leads to Safer Opioid
Prescribing 165
10.2 Balancing Safe Opioid Prescribing with Access to Pain
Management Among Patients with Comorbid Depression 166
10.3 Care Delivery Models to Increase Safe Opioid Prescribing
for Complex Patients with Comorbid Pain and Psychiatric
Conditions 167
10.4 Investing to End the Opioid Epidemic 171

Index 175

Acknowledgments

The editors thank Scott Secrest for his contributions to proofreading and formatting this work.

List of Abbreviations and Acronyms

ACC	Anterior Cingulated Cortex
ACT	Acceptance and Commitment Therapy
ACTH	Adrenocorticotropic Hormone
ANS	Autonomic Nervous System
BD	Bipolar Disorder
BIPOC	Black, Indigenous, and People of Color
CBT	Cognitive Behavioral Therapy
CI	Confidence Interval
CONSORT	Consortium to Study Opioid Risks and Trends
CPOD	Complex Persistent Opioid Dependence
CPT	Current Procedural Terminology
DOR	Delta Opioid Receptor(s)
EAET	Emotional Awareness and Expression Therapy
fMRI	Functional Magnetic Resonance Imaging
HCSRN	Healthcare Systems Research Network
HPA	Hypothalamic Pituitary Adrenal (Axis)
HR	Hazard Ratio
ICD	International Classification of Diseases
IPTW	Inverse Probability of Treatment Weights
KOR	Kappa Opioid Receptor(s)
LOPFC	Lateral Orbital Prefrontal Cortex
LTOT	Long-Term Opioid Therapy
MDvc	Ventral-Caudal Part of the Medial Dorsal Nucleus
MME	Morphine Milligram Equivalents (dose)
MOR	Mu Opioid Receptor(s)
MRI	Magnetic Resonance Imaging
NOP	Nociception/Orphanin FQ Receptors
OICP	Opioid-Induced Chronic Pain Syndrome
OR	Odds Ratio
OUD	Opioid Use Disorder
PAG	Periaqueductal Gray
PCL	PTSD Checklist
PFC	Prefrontal Cortex
PHQ-8	Personal Health Questionnaire 8-item Depression Scale
PNE	Pain Neuroscience Education

xiv LIST OF ABBREVIATIONS AND ACRONYMS

POINT	Pain and Opioids in Treatment Study
PROMIS	Patient-Reported Outcomes Measurement Information System
PRT	Pain Reprocessing Therapy
PS	Propensity Score
PTSD	Post-Traumatic Stress Disorder
RCT	Randomized Control Trial
SCID	Structured Clinical Interview for DSM Disorders
SD	Standard Deviation
SDOH	Social Determinants of Health
SSDOH	Social and Structural Determinants of Health
SUD	Substance Use Disorder
TRD	Treatment Refractory Depression
VHA	Veterans Health Administration
VMPFC	Ventromedial Prefrontal Cortex
VMpo	Posterior Ventral-Medial Nucleus of the Thalamus

List of Contributors

Matthew J. Bair, MD, MS, is Professor of Medicine, Indiana University School of Medicine, Indianapolis, US; Richard L. Roudebush VA Medical Center, Indianapolis, US; Regenstrief Institute, Indianapolis, US.

Jane C. Ballantyne, MD, FRCA, is Professor of Anesthesiology and Pain Medicine at the University of Washington, Seattle, Washington, US.

William C. Becker, MD, is Professor, General Internal Medicine, Yale School of Medicine, US.

Jennifer K. Bello-Kottenstette, MD, MS, is Associate Professor, Family and Community Medicine, Saint Louis University School of Medicine, St. Louis, US.

Travis I. Lovejoy, PhD, MPH, is Professor, Department of Psychiatry, Oregon Health & Science University, Portland, US.

Ajay Manhapra, MD, is a Lecturer at, the Department of Psychiatry, Yale School of Medicine, New Haven, CT, and an Assistant Professor at, the Departments of Psychiatry and Physical Medicine and Rehabilitation, Eastern Virginia Medical School, Norfolk, US.

Lisa R. Miller-Matero, PhD, ABPP, is Associate Scientist, Behavioral Health and Center for Health Policy and Health Services Research, Henry Ford Health, Detroit, US.

Ashli A. Owen-Smith, PhD, SM, is an Associate Professor in the School of Public Health, Georgia State University and Affiliate Investigator Kaiser Permanente Georgia, Atlanta, US.

Geoffrey Panjeton, MD, is an Assistant Professor in the Department of Anesthesiology and Critical Care Faculty member, Saint Louis University, St. Louis, US.

Hess Amir Panjeton, MD, is Assistant Professor of Anesthesiology and Pain Medicine, Washington University School of Medicine, Saint Louis, US.

Robert Rosenheck, MD, is Professor of Psychiatry, Epidemiology and Public Health, and the Child Study Center, Yale Medical School, New Haven, US.

Fred Rottnek, MD, is Director of Community Medicine, Program Director of the Addiction Medicine Fellowship, SSM Health/Saint Louis University, St. Louis, US.

Joanne Salas, MPH, is Director of Applied Research & Analytics, Biostatistics Core of the Advanced Health Data (AHEAD) Institute, Saint Louis University, Saint Louis, US.

xvi LIST OF CONTRIBUTORS

Jeffrey F. Scherrer, PhD, is Professor in the Department of Psychiatry and Behavioral Neuroscience and Vice-Chair for Research and Professor in the Department of Family and Community Medicine and dually appointed Professor in the Department of Psychiatry and Behavioral Neuroscience at Saint Louis University School of Medicine, Missouri, US.

Mark D. Sullivan, MD, PhD, is Professor, Psychiatry and Behavioral Sciences, UW, Seattle, US.

Belle Zaccari, PsyD, is Affiliate Investigator, Center to Improve Veteran Involvement in Care, VA Portland Health Care System, Portland, US; Oregon Health & Science University, Portland, US.

1

Overview and Purpose

Jeffrey F. Scherrer and Jane C. Ballantyne

1.1 Introduction

Opioid prescribing rates peaked in the United States in 2012. Although opioid prescribing in the United States has moderated somewhat,[1] the peak of prescribing left a legacy of patients struggling with opioid dependence. Worse still, there is little doubt that the prescription opioid epidemic continues to contribute to subsequent waves of the U.S. opioid epidemic involving heroin and, later, fentanyl. Much attention is currently focused on the fourth wave of the opioid epidemic, characterized by fentanyl and polydrug abuse.[2] However, minimal progress has been made in reducing prescription opioid overdose deaths. Since 2016, the prevalence of annual drug overdoses involving prescription opioids has remained stable, with 15,000–17,000 overdose deaths per year attributed to prescription opioids.[2] More than 140 million opioid prescriptions were written in 2020, which is sufficient to provide a prescription to 70% of the adult U.S. population. Unfortunately, patients with psychiatric disorders who are at risk for poor outcomes, such as opioid misuse, receive more than 50% of these prescriptions.[3] The prescription opioid epidemic continues to disproportionately impact patients with comorbid pain and mental illness.[4]

This book focuses on a well-recognized clinical and research challenge—the tripartite relationships between pain, long-term prescription opioid use, and psychiatric disorders, particularly depression. By bringing together contributions from neuroscience, pain psychiatry, clinical epidemiology, pharmacoepidemiology, clinical trials, and research on social determinants of health, *Pain, the Opioid Epidemic and Depression* integrates currently siloed areas of investigation and clinical knowledge. As a whole, this work explains the neurophysiology, epidemiology, clinical implications, and social determinants that maintain the pain-depression-opioid tripartite. Our intention is to offer a comprehensive understanding of the central role of depression in the opioid epidemic while also considering the

Jeffrey F. Scherrer and Jane C. Ballantyne, *Overview and Purpose* In: *Pain, the Opioid Epidemic, & Depression.*
Edited by: Jeffrey F. Scherrer & Jane C. Ballantyne, Oxford University Press. © Oxford University Press 2024.
DOI: 10.1093/9780197675250.003.0001

impact of other psychiatric disorders and social determinants of health that contribute to pain management and prescription opioid outcomes. By taking a multidisciplinary approach to compiling what is known about the relationships between pain, prescription opioids, depression, and other psychiatric disorders, this work provides a valuable resource for researchers and clinicians who encounter chronic pain and comorbid mood disorders.

1.2 Chapter Overview

1.2.1 Chapter 2: Neurophysiology of Pain, Depression, and Exogenous Opioids

To better understand the epidemiology and clinical implications of the pain-depression-opioid tripartite, it is necessary to establish the biological relationships between pain and depression, the endogenous opioid system, and the physiological basis for a relationship between prescription opioid use and risk for depression and other adverse mental health outcomes. In Chapter 2, Panjeton and Panjeton discuss biological mechanisms underlying the pain-depression-opioid tripartite and review neuroanatomical changes related to opioid use and how these alterations may contribute to depression and low mood.

1.2.2 Chapter 3: Pain and Depression as Homeostatic Emotion

Chapter 3 provides an in-depth evaluation of pain as both a sensation and an emotion that informs us about our body's integrity. Pain motivates protection of the organism. Sullivan explains how anxiety can also be understood as an emotional state that precipitates behaviors related to reducing perceived danger in one's environment. This definition also fits depression, which could be conceptualized as a general aversive response to the environment. There are common brain structures that both increase vulnerability and are impacted by pain chronicity and negative moods. New therapeutic approaches open up in the context of chronic pain, anxiety, and depression as protective responses to one's environment. Treatments that reduce perceived threats could benefit pain, mood disorder, and the need for chronic prescription opioid use. For some patients, particularly those with mood disorders, non-opioid pain treatments will need to address the pharmacologically induced sense of safety that is part of opioid-induced euphoria.

1.2.3 Chapter 4: Prescription Opioid Use and Risk of Depression and Worsening Mental Health

Depression appears to sustain long-term prescription opioid use and complicates pain management. Depression may arise and existing depression may worsen following long-term opioid therapy (LTOT). Among those with existing depression, long-term compared to short-term opioid use may worsen mood and complicate depression treatment. Chapter 4 offers a critical review of the existing evidence for and against a causal relationship between characteristics of prescription opioid use, such as length of use and morphine equivalent dose, and risk of new-onset and worsening depression.

1.2.4 Chapter 5: Depression and Pain: Bidirectional Relationship and Changes with Psychological Treatment

Depression has a bidirectional relationship with pain. As depression worsens, pain severity and pain-related functional interference increase, and as pain increases, the severity of depression escalates. This has led to the development of psychotherapeutic interventions that target both depression and pain in tandem. These therapies and the logic behind their efficacy are discussed in Chapter 5. Therapies for reducing opioid use are also covered. Therapies that can reduce opioid use and improve pain-related functioning may be followed by improvement in depression and lower risk for new-onset depression. The unique challenges faced by providers and patients with co-morbid pain, depression, and opioid use are reviewed, and opportunities, such as integrated primary care/behavioral health may increase access to needed care for these complex patients. Last, Miller-Matero comments on future directions and policy changes needed to improve access to psychological treatments for pain, mood disorders, and chronic prescription opioid use.

4   JEFFREY F. SCHERRER AND JANE C. BALLANTYNE

1.2.5 Chapter 6: Other Psychiatric Disorders, Psychosocial Factors, Sleep, and Pain

Depression is the most well-studied of the psychiatric disorders comorbid with pain and prescription opioid use. However, other forms of mental illness, such as anxiety disorders, are also more common among persons with chronic pain and among patients receiving long-term prescription opioid therapy. Chapter 6 reviews the evidence for associations between anxiety disorders, posttraumatic stress disorder, bipolar disorder, and schizophrenia with pain and prescription opioid use. This chapter covers the research evidence for these associations and discusses the clinical relevance of comorbid psychiatric disorders on pain management and prescription opioid therapy. The role of sleep disturbance in the interrelationships between chronic pain, comorbid psychiatric disorders, and prescription opioid use is discussed.

1.2.6 Chapter 7: The Impact of Social and Built Determinants on Depression, Prescription Opioid Use, Opioid Misuse, and Opioid Use Disorder

As with other aspects of health, pain, prescription opioid use, and depression are impacted by social determinants of health. Social determinants include employment, housing and food security, health literacy, childhood environment, race and racism, social cohesion, insurance, and access to care. Built environmental determinants include neighborhood crime and violence, housing quality, access to healthy foods and transportation, and internet connectivity. In Chapter 7, Rottnek and Bello-Kottenstette describe how these factors contribute to pain, depression, prescription opioid use, and opioid use disorder, and they explain how differences in education, access to care, health literacy, etc. can lead to health disparities and adverse pain, opioid, and mental health outcomes.

1.2.7 Chapter 8: Opioid Taper and Complex Prescription Opioid Dependence: The Role of Depression and Distress

Opioid taper may be appropriate for some patients with non-cancer pain when the risk of remaining on prescription opioids outweighs the benefits.

For patients with depression and other mental illnesses, tapers can be difficult and clinically destabilizing. Some patients are unable to taper without experiencing extreme distress. In these cases, offering buprenorphine is an option. Increasingly, it is recognized that prescription opioid dependence may require buprenorphine treatment even when classical addiction is not present. Chapter 8 discusses the characteristics of prescription opioid dependence and complex persistent opioid dependence (CPOD), which is an emerging concept in pain management and opioid dependence. Depression symptoms can be elicited during an opioid taper and may be a key component of CPOD. Innovative treatment modalities, such as interdisciplinary pain management clinics, have been developed to help this complex patient population. In Chapter 8, future directions for research are discussed, including a need for studies that can identify patient characteristics associated with better opioid taper outcomes.

1.2.8 Chapter 9: Potential Role for Buprenorphine in the Management of Comorbid Depression Among People with Chronic Pain and Long-Term Opioid Therapy Dependence

Chapter 9 explores emerging evidence regarding buprenorphine's antidepressant effects. Buprenorphine is increasingly prescribed as a less risky option for patients receiving LTOT and for treatment of opioid dependence. Buprenorphine may have antidepressant effects and should be explored as a therapy for complex patients with comorbid pain, depression, and LTOT. Manhapra and colleagues review the history of opioids as antidepressants and discuss the use of buprenorphine as a safer alternative compared to traditional prescription opioids for analgesia. Buprenorphine's antidepressant effects appear to be partly related to improved function and clinical stabilization. Buprenorphine with behavior modification may be an ideal medication for treating comorbid pain, depression, and opioid dependence.

1.3 Key Concepts to Assist Readers

The following section offers definitions for key concepts used throughout this book.

1.3.1 Acute and Chronic Pain

Pain is "an unpleasant sensory and emotional experience associated with or resembling that associated with, actual or potential tissue damage."[5] Pain is subjective and influenced by psychological, social, and physiological factors.[5] Acute pain lasts up to 7 days, with persistence to 30 days not uncommon.[6] "Chronic pain is pain that lasts or recurs longer than 3 months."[7] When unrelated to cancer or cancer treatment, it is considered chronic non-cancer pain. Subtypes of acute and chronic pain are frequently defined by the source of pain, such as musculoskeletal and neuropathic pain. The cause or source of acute pain is more often known as compared to chronic pain. In chronic pain, the biological cause of pain is frequently unknown.

1.3.2 Prescription Opioid Measures

Types of opioids prescribed for non-cancer pain include codeine, dihydrocodeine, fentanyl, hydrocodone, hydromorphone, levorphanol, meperidine, methadone, morphine, oxycodone, oxymorphone, pentazocine, tapentadol, tramadol, and buprenorphine.

Many opioid medications are available in short-acting and long-acting formulations. The Drug Enforcement Agency classifies most opioids as Schedule II medications, which have a high abuse potential.[8] Buprenorphine is a Schedule III opioid with less abuse potential than Schedule II drugs. Tramadol is a Schedule IV opioid with a lower abuse potential.

Duration, dose, and frequency of opioid use have all been studied as both exposures and outcomes in pharmacoepidemiologic studies. Duration is typically measured by counting the number of months a patient had a prescription opioid available. However, this does not necessarily mean that patients used an opioid daily. Some patients have prescriptions for dosing several times a day, while others are prescribed for use as needed. The risk for physiological dependence increases with more frequent opioid use, and frequency of opioid use is another prescription opioid characteristic associated with an increased risk of depression.

Dose can be measured as maximum dose reached during a new opioid use period, average or median dose, or total cumulative amount of opioid consumed. Because each opioid differs in potency, dose is standardized by computing the morphine milligram equivalent (MME). For example, 1 mg of hydrocodone converts to 1 mg of morphine, 1 mg of codeine equals 0.15 mg of morphine, and 1 mg of oxycodone equals 1.5 mg of morphine. The U.S. Centers for Disease Control (CDC) 2016 guideline for prescribing opioids for pain suggested a safe dose should not exceed 90 MME a day[9]; however, the 2022 update to these guidelines emphasizes prescribing at the lowest effective dose.[10] Dose is sometimes modeled as a continuous variable and at other times it is categorized and may be based on policy relevant thresholds. For instance, shortly after the 2016 CDC guideline was published, research on opioid dose would likely use a 90 MME threshold as a way to define a high dose.

The 2022 revised CDC guidelines advise prescribing for the duration that pain is severe enough to require opioids, and reevaluation is suggested when patients require more than 1 month of opioid therapy. Yet existing literature is based on traditional research approaches that have defined chronic opioid use as having a duration of more than 90 days or according to the Consortium to Study Opioid Risks and Trends (CONSORT) definition. CONSORT defines LTOT as a period of opioid use of 90 days, during which the patient had a 120-day supply or greater or 10+ opioid prescriptions dispensed within a 12-month period.

Another important consideration when studying prescription opioid use is whether patients are prevalent users or are starting a new period of prescription opioid use. The most accurate measures of dose and duration are obtained when using a "new user" study design in which patients are enrolled in a cohort when starting a new period of prescription opioid use. A study that follows patients who are existing opioid users at baseline either relies on self-report or would be unable to measure how long patients have been prescription opioid users.

1.4 Overview of the Non-Cancer Pain, Opioid Epidemic, and Depression Tripartite

Chronic pain is a leading cause of disability and poor quality of life. Based on national survey data from 2019, 50.2 million adults (approximately 25%) in the United States report pain on most or every day of the week over the past 3 months.[11] Having chronic pain is associated with a two- to fivefold increased risk of depression.[12] In both the United States and elsewhere, research indicates that depression is a risk factor for chronic pain, but chronic pain can also contribute to new-onset depression.[13] Results from the Stepped Care for Affective Disorders and Musculoskeletal Pain (SCAMP) study indicated that, over a 12-month period, a bidirectional association between severity of pain and depression was observed.[14] When pain severity increased, depression worsened; and, when depression worsened, pain severity increased. Decreasing severity in one condition was followed by improvement in the other. Depression also has a bidirectional association with prescription opioid use and is clearly a key factor in the opioid epidemic.

1.4.1 A Brief Overview of the U.S. Opioid Epidemic

The U.S. opioid epidemic is characterized by four waves. The first wave followed publication of limited and potentially flawed data suggesting addiction rarely occurred among patients taking opioids for pain.[15] This led to marketing of some opioids as having little to no abuse risk.[15] This occurred in the 1990s and followed on the heels of medical societies, the Veterans Health Administration, and other groups promoting the patient's right to pain relief.[16] The 1990s saw the shift from prescribing opioids only for cancer pain to routine use for non-cancer pain.[15] At the time, the pendulum swing went from a clinical setting in which opioids were rarely prescribed for non-cancer pain to liberal prescribing for non-cancer pain in primary care and not just by pain specialists.[15]

The first wave of the opioid epidemic peaked when prescribing rates reached a high in 2012.[15,16] The second wave was characterized by rapid escalation in heroin overdose deaths. The third wave began in 2013, with increasing overdose rates involving fentanyl and other synthetic opioids. The fourth wave, with an onset in the midst of the COVID-19 pandemic, has seen a rise in overdoses involving opioids and polydrug use, particularly stimulants.[15,16]

This volume focuses on long-term prescription opioid use in the context of non-cancer pain and depression. Even though the opioid epidemic has shifted toward non-prescribed fentanyl and polydrug use, this volume is still relevant to the opioid epidemic because there has been no meaningful decline in overdose deaths involving prescription opioids since 2010. The fourth wave of the epidemic has also been accompanied by highly restricted access to opioid analgesics and forced opioid tapering, which has been associated with clinical destabilization, worsening mood, and overdose.[16] The lack of progress in reducing prescription opioid-related overdoses during a time when opioid prescribing has steadily declined (44% decrease in prescribing rates from 2011 to 2019)[16] might be explained by the fact that patients with risk factors for adverse opioid outcomes remain more likely than those without risk factors to be prescribed high-potency and higher abuse potential opioids.[4] While the prescribing rate and dose of prescriptions has declined, the number of prescriptions written for 30 days or more and the days supply per prescription has increased.[1,17] This may contribute to sustaining the mutually reinforcing relationships between pain, opioids, and depression.

1.4.2 Depression and Prescription Opioids

A recent systematic review of psychiatric disorders, chronic pain, and opioid use supports the conclusion that psychiatric comorbidity is associated with increased problem opioid use; greater risk for opioid misuse, abuse, and dependence; more severe opioid craving and worse opioid outcomes; and worse pain interference with daily activities.[12,18] This association is most robust for anxiety and depression.[12,18] Depression is associated with increased non-medical opioid use, such that patients use opioids to treat conditions other than pain (e.g., anxiety or sleep) and take more opioids than prescribed.[12] There is evidence that patients with anxiety and depression experience less analgesia following opioid consumption.[12,18] Fear of anxiety-related physical sensations and catastrophizing in response to pain among those with depression partly explain these associations and likely contribute to seeking opioids.[18] Nationally representative to the United States, analyses of Medical Expenditure Panel Survey data revealed that those with a mental disorder, compared to those without, were more than twice as likely to use prescription opioids after controlling for demographics, access to care, self-reported physical functioning, and substance use disorder.[3] Most striking, more than half of all adult opioid prescriptions are written for the 16% of the U.S. adult population with an active mental illness.[3]

Greater odds of receiving an opioid, higher doses, and faster dose escalation have been observed in patients with chronic non-cancer pain who have, versus do not have, either a mental health diagnosis or substance use disorder.[12,19] Mood disorders are associated with twice the likelihood of transitioning from short-term to long-term opioid use,[20] and depression increases risk for overuse and non-medical prescription opioid use.[20]

1.5 Clinical and Public Health Relevance

Depression has been established as a risk for adverse prescription opioid outcomes, and LTOT and daily or near daily opioid use are risk factors for depression. Despite this knowledge, there has been little change in clinical practice to address the bidirectional relationship between prescription opioids and depression. The revised 2022 CDC prescribing guidelines recommend screening for "depression and mental health conditions" prior to initiating LTOT. The guidelines do not discuss screening for other psychiatric conditions, such as anxiety disorders. The CDC prescribing guidelines do not mention whether treatment and improvement in depression or in other psychiatric conditions reduce risk for adverse opioid outcomes. Last, despite evidence that LTOT worsens mood,[21,22] there is no guidance on repeat monitoring for mental illness during LTOT.

As illustrated in Figure 1.1, pain, depression, and prescription opioid use may have mutually reinforcing relationships. Pain contributes to worsening depression, and depression contributes to increased odds of long-term prescription opioid use that, in turn, exacerbates risk for new or recurring depressive episodes. By treating depression and other psychiatric disorders to remission, it may be possible to break the cycle shown in Figure 1.1.

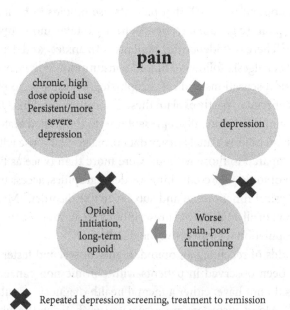

Figure 1.1 Stopping the pain, depression, opioid cycle.

OVERVIEW AND PURPOSE 11

Prescribing guidelines should emphasize the importance of mental health treatment. Research is needed to determine if remitted depression, improved mood, and improvement in other psychiatric disorders are followed by shorter, lower-dose prescription opioid use. The evidence presented in this volume establishes the rationale for such guideline revisions and offers novel ideas on delivering integrated healthcare to treat the whole patient, not just pain symptoms.

References

1. Bohnert ASB, Guy GP, Jr., Losby JL. Opioid prescribing in the United States before and after the Centers for Disease Control and Prevention's 2016 Opioid Guideline. *Ann Intern Med.* 2018;169(6):367–375.
2. Centers for Disease Control and Prevention. Prescription opioid overdose death maps. https://www.cdc.gov/drugoverdose/deaths/prescription/maps.html. Accessed Feb. 15, 2023.
3. Davis MA, Lin LA, Liu H, Sites BD. Prescription opioid use among adults with mental health disorders in the United States. *J Am Board Fam Med.* 2017;30(4):407–417.
4. Scherrer JF, Tucker J, Salas J, Zhang Z, Grucza R. Comparison of opioids prescribed for patients at risk for opioid misuse before and after publication of the Centers for Disease Control and Prevention's Opioid Prescribing Guidelines. *JAMA Network Open.* 2020;3(12):e2027481.
5. Raja SN, Carr DB, Cohen M, et al. The revised International Association for the Study of Pain definition of pain: Concepts, challenges, and compromises. *Pain.* 2020;161(9):1976–1982.
6. Kent ML, Tighe PJ, Belfer I, et al. The ACTTION-APS-AAPM Pain Taxonomy (AAAPT) multidimensional approach to classifying acute pain conditions. *J Pain.* 2017;18(5):479–489.
7. Treede RD, Rief W, Barke A, et al. Chronic pain as a symptom or a disease: The IASP classification of chronic pain for the International Classification of Diseases (ICD-11). *Pain.* 2019;160(1):19–27.
8. U.S. Department of Justice, Drug Enforcement Administration. *Drugs of Abuse: A DEA Resource Guide.* 2017.
9. Dowell D, Haegerich TM, Chou R. CDC Guideline for Prescribing Opioids for Chronic Pain: United States, 2016. *JAMA.* 2016;315(15):1624–1645.
10. Centers for Disease Control and Prevention. CDC's Clinical Practice Guideline for Prescribing Opioids for Pain. https://www.cdc.gov/opioids/healthcare-professionals/prescribing/guideline/index.html?s_cid=DOP_Clinician_Search_Paid_001&gclid=EAIaIQobChMI3NXrwIKZgQMVwvCUCR2MggTbEAAYASAAEgK-RPD_BwE.Accessed Sep. 7, 2023.
11. Yong RJ, Mullins PM, Bhattacharyya N. Prevalence of chronic pain among adults in the United States. *Pain.* 2022;163(2):e328–e332.
12. Howe CQ, Sullivan MD. The missing "P" in pain management: How the current opioid epidemic highlights the need for psychiatric services in chronic pain care. *General Hospital Psychiatry.* 2014;36(1):99–104.
13. Kroenke K, Bair MJ, Damush TM, et al. Optimized antidepressant therapy and pain self-management in primary care patients with depression and musculoskeletal pain: A randomized controlled trial. *JAMA.* 2009;301(20):2099–2110.

14. Kroenke K, Wu J, Bair MJ, Krebs EE, Damush TM, Tu W. Reciprocal relationship between pain and depression: A 12-month longitudinal analysis in primary care. *J Pain.* 2011;12:964–973.
15. Bernard SA, Chelminski PR, Ives TJ, Ranapurwala SI. Management of pain in the United States: A brief history and implications for the opioid epidemic. *Health Serv Insights.* 2018;11:1178632918819440.
16. Manchikanti L, Singh VM, Staats PS, et al. Fourth wave of opioid (illicit drug) overdose deaths and diminishing access to prescription opioids and interventional techniques: Cause and effect. *Pain Physician.* 2022;25(2):97–124.
17. Guy GP, Jr., Zhang K, Schieber LZ, Young R, Dowell D. County-level opioid prescribing in the United States, 2015 and 2017. *JAMA Intern Med.* 2019;179(4):574–576.
18. van Rijswijk SM, van Beek M, Schoof GM, Schene AH, Steegers M, Schellekens AF. Iatrogenic opioid use disorder, chronic pain and psychiatric comorbidity: A systematic review. *Gen Hosp Psychiatry.* 2019;59:37–50.
19. Edlund MJ, Martin BC, Fan MY, Devries A, Braden JB, Sullivan MD. Risks for opioid abuse and dependence among recipients of chronic opioid therapy: results from the TROUP study. *Drug Alcohol Depend.* 2010;112(1–2):90–98.
20. Sullivan MD. Why does depression promote long-term opioid use? *Pain.* 2016;157(11):2395–2396.
21. Scherrer JF, Svrakic DM, Freedland KE, et al. Prescription opioid analgesics increase the risk of depression. *J Gen Intern Med.* 2014;29(3):491–499.
22. Scherrer JF, Salas J, Copeland LA, et al. Prescription opioid duration, dose, and increased risk of depression in 3 large patient populations. *Ann Fam Med.* 2016;14:54–62.

2

Neurophysiology of Pain, Depression, and Exogenous Opioids

Geoffrey Panjeton and Hess Amir Panjeton

2.1 Introduction

Pain is defined by an integration of negative sensory and emotional-affective perceptions. The purpose of this experience is to alert to and provide a protective mechanism against a potentially harmful stimulus. However, with chronicity and prolonged exposure to certain stimuli, this signaling can be maladaptive and result in a variety of harmful consequences. Depression is a commonly exhibited comorbidity in patients experiencing chronic pain. The connection between pain and depression, although clinically very common and apparent, can be difficult to dissect. Chronic pain has been shown to be a major obstacle in the full remission of symptoms of a clinically depressed patient.[1] The majority of patients suffering from depression continued to have residual symptoms when they were concurrently experiencing some form of chronic pain.[1]

2.2 Neurophysiological Mechanisms Underlying Comorbid Pain and Depression

Although pain and depression have long been recognized as closely intertwined conditions, the relationship underlying the two is not fully understood. Dersh and colleagues presented five hypotheses that have been proposed in the literature as plausible explanations of the underlying relationship between pain and depression.[2] These are (1) the consequence hypothesis, (2) the cognitive behavioral mediation hypothesis, (3) the scar hypothesis, (4) the diathesis-stress model, and (5) the common pathogenetic mechanisms hypothesis.

Geoffrey Panjeton and Hess Amir Panjeton, *Neurophysiology of Pain, Depression, and Exogenous Opioids* In: *Pain, the Opioid Epidemic, & Depression*. Edited by: Jeffrey F. Scherrer & Jane C. Ballantyne, Oxford University Press.
© Oxford University Press 2024. DOI: 10.1093/9780197675250.003.0002

The *consequence hypothesis* describes depression as a consequence of pain development, implicating pain as a primary condition and depression as a secondary or consequent effect. The *cognitive behavioral mediation hypothesis* posits that specific cognitions may mediate the relationship between depression and pain. Specifically, negative thoughts and beliefs surrounding pain may predispose an individual to developing depression in the presence of chronic pain. The *scar hypothesis* suggests that the presence of episodic depression in the pre-pain state may lead to an increased propensity to developing depression following the onset of pain.[2] According to this theory, prior episodes of depression may leave an individual more vulnerable to depression in the presence of pain.[2] The *diathesis-stress model* refers to an underlying psychological diathesis, or predisposition, that is semi-dormant prior to the onset of pain and is then made manifest by the stress related to the chronic pain state. This theory suggests that certain individuals may have an underlying vulnerability to psychopathology prior to the onset of chronic pain and that the stress of the chronic pain state can exacerbate these symptoms.

Finally, the *common pathogenetic mechanisms hypothesis*, which is the focus of the ensuing chapter, describes the similarities between the underlying physiology and neurotransmitters involved in the development and mediation of depression and pain, namely serotonin and norepinephrine.[2] This theory suggests that depression and pain are related due to shared underlying mechanisms in the brain.[2]

2.3 Common Underlying Physiology

To begin understanding the connection between pain and depression, one need only look to the specific neurotransmitters involved in both processes. Norepinephrine and serotonin are often implicated in the development of depression. From a biochemical perspective an imbalance or deficiency in norepinephrine, serotonin, and dopamine have been proposed as a cause of depression.[3] Norepinephrine and serotonin have also been identified as key mediators in the endogenous analgesic mechanism of the descending pain pathway.[4] Therefore, patients with imbalances in their serotonin and norepinephrine systems may experience heightened pain due to ineffective modulation in the descending pathways.[5]

The hypothalamic-pituitary-adrenal (HPA) axis is also implicated in the relationship between pain and depression. Dysfunction at the HPA axis is often identified in patients with depression and manifested by elevated adrenocorticotropic hormone and cortisol plasma concentrates.[5] The typical role of the HPA axis is to mediate the body's response to a stressful stimulus. The effect of stress and dysregulation of the HPA axis leads to high concentrations of cortisol in depressed individuals.[1] HPA axis hyperactivity reduces sensitivity to the inhibitory effects of the glucocorticoid dexamethasone on the production of adrenocorticotropic hormone (ACTH) and cortisol during the dexamethasone suppression test.[1] Furthermore, glucocorticoid receptor downregulation is a likely cause of HPA axis dysregulation in depressed individuals.[1] In the chronic pain state, the HPA axis is influenced by the release of cytokines such as interleukin-1 or interleukin-6 which in turn cause increased ACTH and corticosteroid levels.[1] The downstream sequela of noxious stimuli and release of these cytokines may also lead to chronic pain conditions like neuropathic pain. In similar chronic pain conditions, monoaminergic neurons in the brainstem, which normally descend to the spinal cord to act as regulators to inhibit nociceptive stimuli, are lost as a result of glucocorticoid-induced monoamine depletion.[1] This loss of monoaminergic tone leads to reduced descending inhibitory drive, which enhances pain sensation in chronic pain sufferers.[1] However, patients in chronic pain states may represent prolonged and continued stress, and this may disrupt this process, resulting in depletion of central serotonin and dysregulation at a variety of other receptors associated with depression.[5]

The main structure involved in pain modulation is the periaqueductal gray (PAG), and it is a connecting point for pathways between the limbic forebrain and midbrain (amygdala, hypothalamus, and frontal neocortex) with the brainstem (pons and medulla).[3] These connections typically include both serotonergic and adrenergic neurons which, in concert with the limbic structures and the PAG, are involved in the affect and attention to peripheral stimuli.[3] In typical circumstances, these systems work to modulate and decrease the intensity of the stimuli; however, in patients with decreased serotonin and norepinephrine, these signals may be intensified.[3] These systems are part of a complex network of communications between cortical structures involved in emotion such as the medial prefrontal cortex, insular, anterior temporal cortex, hypothalamus, and amygdala, with the brainstem structures involved in pain modulation, like the PAG.[3]

Support for some of these effects, such as the effect of the amygdala and the anterior cingulate cortex on pain modulation, has been provided by functional magnetic resonance imaging (fMRI) studies.[5] In particular, the medial temporal lobe of the amygdala has been reported to house a cluster of nuclei involved in both pain and negative affective states.[5] In addition to the amygdala, the anterior cingulated cortex (ACC), hippocampus, and most especially the prefrontal cortex (PFC), are involved in the neuropathology of depression.[1] These structures demonstrate significant atrophy in patients with depression. In fMRI studies of these individuals with depression, there appears to be a decreased activation in areas of the PFC and increased activation of the limbic system (e.g., amygdala, hippocampus).[1] Specifically, the ventromedial prefrontal cortex (VMPFC) and the lateral orbital prefrontal cortex (LOPFC) within the PFC exhibit the greatest decreases in metabolism among people with depression.[1] Consequently, similar areas of the PFC implicated in depression play a role in the modulation of pain. In both chronic pain and depression, there appears to be a link associated with increased limbic activity resulting in the propagation of symptoms of depression and pain among patients with both of these comorbidities.[1] Depression is typically correlated with increased activity in the amygdala, and the relationship between aberrant functioning of the amygdala and negative affective states is well established.[5] The amygdala plays a bidirectional role in pain processing, with the ability to inhibit or enhance the pain signal.[5] The increased activity noted in negative affective states may stimulate the pain-facilitating pathways.[5] Although there is some conflicting literature related to the nature of the change in activity in the amygdala in response to pain, the evidence suggests that the amygdala plays a critical role in the relationship between pain and depression.[5]

2.4 The Role of Opioid Medications on the Link Between Pain and Depression

Opioid medications exert their effect through opioid receptors, which are a type of G-protein coupled receptors and are categorized as mu (MOR), kappa (KOR), and delta (DOR).[6] Endogenous opioid substances are present throughout the central and peripheral nervous systems, such as beta-endorphin, enkephalins, and dynorphins.[6] Opioid peptides and receptors are involved in a number of physiological activities including pain processing, stress response, respiration, gastrointestinal motility, endocrine, and immune functions.[6] Each of the opioid receptors has been implicated in reward processing, with subsequent effects on mood. Specifically, mice models with genetic deletions of MOR and DOR have revealed behaviors resembling anxiety and depression, suggesting these opioid receptors may play a role in regulating emotional responses.[6] Drawing from addiction research, strong evidence demonstrates the influence of MOR and DOR on dopamine release in the nucleus accumbens.[6] KOR are expressed on the presynaptic terminals of dopamine neurons in the nucleus accumbens and may play a role in decreasing dopamine secretion, resulting in depressed mood.[6] KOR activity may be involved in mediating the effects of stressful states, and this has been associated with depressive phenotypes.[7,8] The effect of this relationship on clinical manifestations of depression requires further investigation.

Beyond the receptors and endogenous peptides, prescription opioids have been shown to contribute to new-onset depression or worsen existing depressive symptoms. Although acute administrations of morphine increase serotonin levels throughout the limbic regions of the brain in rats and mice, chronic morphine administration led to decreased serotonin activity upon interruption of treatment and during withdrawal.[6] The decrease in serotonin activity was a result of a compensatory upregulation of the gamma aminobutyric acid (GABA)ergic tone on the serotonin neurons in the presence of the chronic morphine administration.[6] Conversely, in the noradrenergic system, acute morphine administration resulted in decreased norepinephrine release in the forebrain, and following cessation of chronic treatment there was a rebound hyperactivity of the noradrenergic system.[6]

These findings suggest that although acute opioid administrations may be euphoric in nature, treatment chronicity may predispose to the development of depression.[6] From a neurobiological perspective, there are specific findings that may set the stage for the increased risk of depression. Chronic morphine administration resulted in adaptations of the serotonin 5-HT_{1A} receptor, and this adaptation has also been established in rodent models of depression.[6] Finally, chronic morphine administration demonstrated structural changes in the hippocampus and dentate gyrus, such as decreased dendritic spine density and decreased neuronal proliferation.[6] These changes demonstrate that prolonged activation of MOR can have deleterious effects on hippocampal plasticity and neurogenesis.[6]

Neuroanatomical changes have also been identified in patients with chronic prescription opioid use, and these may be related to emotional dysregulation and aberrant reward processing. As soon as 1 month following daily morphine use, dose-dependent neuroplastic changes with resulting volumetric changes are noticed in several brain regions.[9] In particular, the amygdala demonstrated reductions in gray matter, and the cingulate and hypothalamus demonstrated increases in gray matter.[9] This finding was also established in patients with significant longstanding prescription opioid dependence when compared with healthy controls.[10] Atrophy in the amygdala is concerning for possibly impairing natural reward processes and its effect on learning processes and behavior patterns.[9] Beyond the structural atrophy, more detailed imaging analysis also demonstrated compromise in the functional connectivity of the amygdala in patients with long-standing opioid dependence.[10] The opioid-dependent patients also demonstrated significantly decreased anisotropy in the axonal pathways of the internal and external capsules and the efferent and afferent pathways of the amygdala.[10] Functional connectivity was compromised in the anterior insula, amygdala, and nucleus accumbens pathways, with the degree of effect correlated to duration of prescription opioid dependence.[10] The negative effects of longstanding opioid use on white matter integrity may be a result of harmful effects of opioids on myelin and other axonal membrane properties because oligodendrocytes express opioid receptors.[10]

Increased gray matter was seen in regions with high MOR density, binding capacity, and strong response to opioid administration.[9] Of note was the increase in the gray matter in the hypothalamus, where opioids can inhibit the function of the HPA axis.[9] This can also manifest inhibitory effects of opioids on the hypothalamic hypocretin system, which may generate depression symptoms such as lethargy and decreased cognition following chronic opioid use.[9] Of great concern in these findings is that they remained stable and persistent even 4 months after opioid cessation, and this may illustrate the long-lasting effects of even brief exposures of consistent opioid use.[9]

2.5 Hedonic Capacity Related to Chronic Opioid Use

Hedonic capacity is related to the ability to feel pleasure when experiencing naturally rewarding stimuli and is a critical component of emotional well-being. There is a neurobiological underpinning that relates these social and emotional experiences with pain receptor mechanisms. When investigating across a variety of substance use disorders, anhedonia was most notable among those with opioid use disorder.[11] At a neuronal level, social isolation demonstrated similar activity as nociceptive circuits in several species, giving depth to the meaning of "emotional pain".[6] Similarly, social behaviors in rodents demonstrated release of endogenous opioid peptides.[6] With chronic opioid use, patients may experience a "reward deficiency" state that may exacerbate the negative effect on their social and hedonic state. The reward-deficient state is aggravated by release of KOR agonist dynorphin which ultimately results in the production of a stress state characterized by release of norepinephrine, corticotropin-releasing factor, vasopressin, hypocretin, and substance P.[12] As time progresses and patients are exposed to opioids for a longer duration, this stress-like response converts the impetus for opioid seeking from seeking pleasure to the negative reinforcement of avoiding hyperalgesia and dysphoria.[13]

2.6 Conclusion

Individuals with long-term opioid use are at increased risk for new-onset depression, recurrent depression, and worsening depression.[13] Although much work remains to be done to better understand the nuances of this relationship, it is clear that there exists a variety of neurobiological interactions and correlated physiology that inextricably pairs the pain and mood perception pathways. Alterations in either of these mechanisms appear to exacerbate pathology in the other, and the resulting clinical manifestation of depression in patients with chronic pain is apparent.

References

1. Boakye PA, Olechowski C, Rashiq S, et al. A critical review of neurobiological factors involved in the interactions between chronic pain, depression, and sleep disruption. *Clin J Pain.* 2016;32(4):327–336.
2. Dersh J, Polatin PB, Gatchel RJ. Chronic pain and psychopathology: Research findings and theoretical considerations. *Psychosom Med.* 2002;64(5):773–786.
3. Bair MJ, Robinson RL, Katon W, Kroenke K. Depression and pain comorbidity: A literature review. *Arch Intern Med.* 2003;163(20):2433–2445.
4. Marks DM, Shah MJ, Patkar AA, Masand PS, Park GY, Pae CU. Serotonin-norepinephrine reuptake inhibitors for pain control: Premise and promise. *Curr Neuropharmacol.* 2009;7(4):331–336.

5. Williams LJ, Jacka FN, Pasco JA, Dodd S, Berk M. Depression and pain: An overview. *Acta Neuropsychiatr.* 2006;18(2):79–87.
6. Lutz PE, Kieffer BL. Opioid receptors: Distinct roles in mood disorders. *Trends Neurosci.* 2013;36(3):195–206.
7. Scherrer JF, Salas J, Copeland LA, et al. Prescription opioid duration, dose, and increased risk of depression in 3 large patient populations. *Ann Fam Med.* 2016;14(1):54–62.
8. Van't Veer A, Carlezon WA, Jr. Role of kappa-opioid receptors in stress and anxiety-related behavior. *Psychopharmacology (Berl).* 2013;229(3):435–452.
9. Younger JW, Chu LF, D'Arcy NT, Trott KE, Jastrzab LE, Mackey SC. Prescription opioid analgesics rapidly change the human brain. *Pain.* 2011;152(8):1803–1810.
10. Upadhyay J, Maleki N, Potter J, et al. Alterations in brain structure and functional connectivity in prescription opioid-dependent patients. *Brain.* 2010;133(Pt 7):2098–2114.
11. Stull SW, Bertz JW, Epstein DH, Bray BC, Lanza ST. Anhedonia and substance use disorders by type, severity, and with mental health disorders. *J Addict Med.* 2022;16(3):e150–e156.
12. Elman I, Borsook D. Common brain mechanisms of chronic pain and addiction. *Neuron.* 2016;89(1):11–36.
13. Bates N, Bello JK, Osazuwa-Peters N, Sullivan MD, Scherrer JF. Depression and long-term prescription opioid use and opioid use disorder: Implications for pain management in cancer. *Curr Treat Options Oncol.* 2022;23(3):348–358.

3

Looking Beyond Tissue Damage

Pain as a Homeostatic Emotion

Mark D. Sullivan

3.1 Introduction

When I burn my finger or sprain my ankle, I look to my damaged body part as the cause of my pain. This pain appears to be providing me information about tissue damage so I can protect this body part from further damage. My pain is localized to the body part with damage so I can direct my protective efforts appropriately. Pain thus appears to be operating similar to touch in providing us information about something that is happening to a specific part of our body.

These intuitive ideas about pain and tissue damage have been reflected in years of scientific pain research. Psychophysical experiments by Don Price and others defined precise mathematical relationships between noxious stimulus intensity and the intensity of pain sensation produced.[1] This is consistent with a distinction introduced by Sherrington, in 1906, between cutaneous exteroceptors activated by objects in the external environment and interoceptors activated by bodily changes in the internal environment, such as the gastrointestinal tract.[2] Price argued that spinal wide dynamic range and nociceptive-specific neurons "function in a coordinated manner to encode the sensory-discriminative features of external nociceptive stimuli."[1]

These ideas about pain being an exteroceptive faculty were carried into the clinical domain through instruments like the McGill Pain Questionnaire, created by Ronald Melzack. This questionnaire famously distinguished between three distinct dimensions of pain experience: sensory-discriminative, affective-emotional, and cognitive-evaluative.[3] Although this questionnaire sought to capture pain as a multidimensional experience, these dimensions were often thought to occur in sequence, with sensory-discriminative features processed before affective-emotional and cognitive-evaluative

Mark D. Sullivan, *Looking Beyond Tissue Damage* In: *Pain, the Opioid Epidemic, & Depression*. Edited by: Jeffrey F. Scherrer & Jane C. Ballantyne, Oxford University Press. © Oxford University Press 2024. DOI: 10.1093/9780197675250.003.0003

22 MARK D. SULLIVAN

features. This serial processing view of pain supported the idea that pain was primarily a sensory phenomenon that prompted an emotional reaction. Subsequent studies by Rainville of the effects of hypnotic suggestion on pain intensity versus pain unpleasantness appeared to support the primacy of the sensory properties of pain.[4] But clinical pain, and especially chronic pain, is only loosely related to the degree of tissue damage and the activity in peripheral nociceptors.

3.2 Alternative View: Pain as Interoceptive Homeostatic Emotion

An alternative view to pain providing information about the external world was proffered by neuroscientist Bud Craig in a series of papers from 2003 to 2013. Craig argued that pain is better understood as an interoceptive homeostatic emotion.[5] Using largely anatomical data, Craig claimed that pain is more similar to temperature, itch, and hunger perception than to touch.[6] In subprimates, a phylogenetically old nociceptive pathway is dominant. Wide dynamic range neurons in lamina V of the dorsal horn of the spinal cord send axons up the lateral spinothalamic pathway into the somatosensory ventro-posterior thalamus and then on to the somatosensory cortex (S_1 and S_{11}). This yields the intensity-related sensorimotor neuronal activity and behavior expected from the exteroceptive model.

But in primates, Craig argues, a new medial spinal pathway exists alongside this older pathway. This new pathway transmits specific interoceptive information from lamina I dorsal horn neurons through the medial thalamus to the insular cortex ("feeling self") and to the anterior cingulate cortex ("behavioral agent"). Specifically, these lamina I neurons project in the crossed lateral spinothalamic tract to the posterior ventral medial nucleus (VMpo) of the thalamus and to the ventral caudal part of the medial dorsal nucleus (MDvc). The VMpo projects a high-resolution, modality-specific sensory representation of the physiological condition of the body in the interoceptive cortex at the dorsal margin of the insula. This area has many receptors for corticotropin-releasing factor, which provides further information about homeostasis and stress. The MDvc integrates lamina I input with brainstem homeostatic activity (transmitted from the parabrachial nucleus and the periaqueductal gray) and produces activity in the limbic motor cortex (anterior cingulate), resulting in behavioral drive (Figure 3.1). These generate the

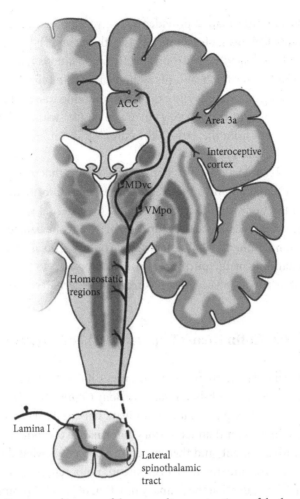

Figure 3.1 Summary diagram of the ascending projections of the lamina I spino-thalamo-cortical system.

Used with permission of Annual Review of Neuroscience Pain Mechanisms: Labeled Lines Versus Convergence in Central Processing A.D. (Bud) Craig Annual Review of Neuroscience 2003;26:1, 1–30 permission conveyed through Copyright Clearance Center, Inc.

feeling and motivation, respectively, that constitute the homeostatic emotion of pain.

What Craig describes here is no less than "the long missing sensory complement of the efferent autonomic nervous system (ANS)." As Walter Cannon contended, the neural processes that maintain an optimal physiological balance (which he called "homeostasis") across body systems must receive modality-specific afferent inputs reporting the condition of the tissues of the body. This information provides not only for homeostatic control, but also for bodily feelings such as hunger, taste, thirst, and shortness of breath. These are all associated with strong affective motivations that promote behavior that maintains the health of the body. By calling these "homeostatic emotions," Craig emphasizes the essential autonomic role of these feelings. These theories are not entirely new but are consistent with the James-Lange theory of emotion from the early 20th century and Antonio Damasio's "somatic marker" hypothesis.[7]

The clinical implication of this homeostatic view is that pain is simultaneously both a sensation and a motivation. It provides information about the integrity of the body, not information about the external world. This view helps explain the variable relationship of pain with tissue damage by placing its production within a global homeostatic context. This is consistent with our understanding of the purpose of pain perception: to preserve the organism, not to provide an accurate picture of the external world.

3.3 Colin Klein's Imperative Theory of Pain

A similar theory of pain can be found in a very different source. In 2015, philosopher Colin Klein published *What The Body Commands: The Imperative Theory of Pain*.[8] He argues that the motivational-emotional component of pain is more important than its sensory-informative component. "All pains have imperative content, and that imperative content is what distinguishes them as pains." An imperative is a command, not a representation or a description. Klein argues that the primary function of pain is to command protective behavior rather than to inform us of tissue damage.

Most sensory experiences, such as visual or auditory sensations, inform us of the outside world, but pain does not. "Ordinary sensations inform but don't necessarily motivate. Pains motivate without informing. That is why pain is unusual." Pain is typically localized in a body part, and this helps direct our protective efforts to that body part. But for many common pains in clinical practice, and for most chronic pains, this localization is not very precise. However, Klein contends, it is precise enough to direct our protective efforts and that satisfies its purpose.

A patient or clinician can investigate the cause of pain, but this does not prove the experience of pain to be a true or false representation. Primary care clinicians have often considered pains without clear association with tissue damage to be unreal, exaggerated, or non-medical pain. There is an extensive literature on "medically unexplained pain" and its association with psychiatric disorders.[9,10] But this concept of unexplained pain assumes that real pain is caused by tissue damage. Clinical pain cannot be proved to be true or false through correlation with imaging or physical exam findings. Patients are understandably offended when clinicians say, "I can't find anything wrong with your back." Yet pain without identifiable tissue damage is a common clinical occurrence.

Clinicians and patients alike assumed that the many abnormalities detected by magnetic resonance imaging (MRI) of the lumbar spine were causing the back pain of patients who obtained these scans in clinical care. Patients appreciated the validation that these imaging studies provided for their pain complaints.[11] Workers' compensation and other disability programs routinely required validation of pain-related disability through association with imaging abnormalities. It was not until 1994, when Jensen et al. published their landmark study, "Magnetic Resonance Imaging of the Lumbar Spine in People Without Back Pain" in the *New England Journal of Medicine* that doubts about the causal role of common degenerative changes in the spine and its discs were validated.[12] Disc bulges and protrusions were found in many people with *no back pain*. This study has been replicated many times, demonstrating that many of the most common findings on spinal MRI often do not cause back pain. In fact, multiple studies have demonstrated that among patients with low back pain (but no red flags for serious systemic illness), early MRI is not associated with better health outcomes but is associated with increased likelihood of disability and its duration.[13,14]

3.4 Pain in the Brain: From Pain Matrix to Salience Network

It has long been recognized that pain perception does not occur in a dedicated single center in the brain. However, it is not that long ago that pain perception was thought to occur in a dedicated but distributed set of brain structures, such as the primary (S_I) and secondary (S_{II}) somatosensory, the cingulate, and the insular cortices, called the "pain matrix," that were found to have activity that correlated with pain intensity reports.[15] However, more recent studies have shown that in many circumstances the activity in this pain matrix matches neither the subjective intensity of pain experienced nor the objective intensity of the nociceptive stimulus.[16]

It has therefore been argued that brain centers specific to pain perception are better considered a multisensory "salience network"[17-19] activated by sensory events of various modalities that indicate or predict a threat to the body's integrity. These threatening events include not only somatosensory nociceptive stimuli but also non-nociceptive visual and auditory stimuli that contribute to the determination of the salience or relevance of input to the organism's survival. Non-nociceptive threatening stimuli may produce a pattern of brain activity nearly identical to that produced by nociceptive stimuli.[20] The activity in the brain areas that respond to nociceptive stimuli is therefore not a reflection of pain intensity but of threat salience. *Salience* is a measure of the importance of the stimulus for the organism and its survival. In moving from stimulus *intensity* to stimulus *salience*, we have begun to synthesize biological *mechanisms* and psychosocial *meanings* in the etiology of pain.

The brain's salience network expands the influences on pain experience from nociception to multisensory indicators of safety or danger and thus offers a pathway by which personal meaning interacts with impersonal nociceptive mechanisms. Legrain et al. explain, "Indeed, salience detectors represent the neural mechanism by which selective attention is captured and oriented towards the most salient stimuli in order to prioritize their processing over background stimuli, to improve their perception and to prompt appropriate action."[21] The salience network integrates internal and external factors—nociception and psychosocial influences on pain—to promote survival. This means, according to Legrain, "that the purpose of pain is not merely to induce and to associate the feeling of unpleasantness to a somatosensory sensation, but it also to warn the body about potential physical threats."

Furthermore, these potential threats are not limited to damage within the body. For example, salience network neurons may respond to visual objects (e.g., a wasp) as they are *approaching* the body, but not when they are *moving away* from the body. Salience detection includes the body *and* the environment within grasping distance. There is a close relationship between visual, proprioceptive, and tactile processing of threats in this near-personal space.

A salience-focused approach means that the brain is changed by events inside and outside of the body. It also helps us understand the variable relationship between pain experience and tissue damage. This variability includes feeling pain in the absence of a noxious stimulus, reporting minimal pain in the setting of major tissue damage, having an "analgesic" response when no analgesic has been administered, or producing no pain relief after administration of a potent analgesic medication. The salience network idea helps explain why psychological trauma that produces no tissue damage can be associated with dramatic increases in pain.[22] If pain arises from danger detection, its truth or falsity is more complicated. Danger is not an objective property of the body.

If pain arises from danger, this also helps explain why pain may persist after tissue healing has been completed. As Klein explains, "Most work on pain assumes that pain serves as a symptom of damage. . . . [But] in ordinary cases pain is not a symptom but part of the cure." This means that pain is not something done to us but is part of the organism's protective response. Pain persists as a protection from danger. This echoes a similar statement from Patrick Wall, one of the creators of the gate control theory of pain, who claimed that pain does not inform to protect, but to motivate recovery.

The presence and intensity of pain are too poorly related to the degree of damage to be considered such a messenger (of damage). Pain is a poor protector against injury since it occurs far too late in the case of sudden injury or very slow damage to provide a useful preventive measure. Instead, it is proposed that pain signals the existence of a body state where recovery and recuperation should be initiated.[23]

Pain commands protective action in a specific way, as a homeostatic sensation. These demands cannot be put off indefinitely. They are not optional parts of one's motivational situation. Severe hunger commands my attention unless something appears that will kill me even more quickly. Furthermore, Klein explains, "homeostatic sensations motivate types of action rather than specific particular actions: eating, drinking, smoking, or scratching." There is both urgency and flexibility in these commands. This flexibility distinguishes homeostatic emotions from classical reflex behavior. Classical reflexes promote an immediate, single, fixed behavior, but homeostatic sensations promote a more flexible and potentially delayed response to restore balance. Klein elaborates:

> Homeostatic sensations thus represent a halfway house between mere reflexes and full agential desires: although they motivate action, they do so in a way that allows for deliberation and other sorts of top-down control. . . . Homeostatic sensations give just the right amount of flexibility: flexibility as to when the homeostatic demand is satisfied and how you satisfy it, but not as to whether you act or what you do to satisfy it. (pp. 16–17)[8]

28 MARK D. SULLIVAN

We often look at pain as a mechanically produced sensation that mandates withdrawal and immobility of the injured body part. But the relation of injury to pain and the relation of pain to behavior is more complicated than this. The pain system is smarter than we often assume. Both the injury–pain relation and the pain–behavior relation are modified to support the survival and the homeostasis of the affected organism.

3.5 The Relation of Pain to Hurt and Suffering

Klein sees pain as having two kinds of motivational force. Its primary motivational force arises from the intrinsic properties of pain. This is the urgent motivation to protect a body part. "*Secondary* motivation, by contrast, includes all motivational states that are properly extrinsic to pain. This includes any mental states that are *caused* by or *directed toward* the sensation of pain. Because secondary motivations are not intrinsic to pain, they can be entirely absent when we feel pain" (p. 45). This means that "suffering is not a feature of pain: it is a response to pain." He points to grief and heartbreak as examples of suffering that are distinct from pain. Catastrophizing, which can accompany chronic pain, is also framed as secondary and more a part of suffering than pain. Klein follows previous pain researchers (like Price) in understanding pain intensity as an intrinsic feature of pain but pain unpleasantness as a secondary property caused by pain. He summarizes: "The point is that the two kinds of motivation have wholly different targets: one motivates actions with respect to the *body*, whereas the other motivates action with respect to a *mental state*" (p. 53). Here is where I must part with Klein's generally excellent account. Ultimately, his account works better for localized nociceptive pain and less well for generalized nociplastic pain. It is in patients with more generalized and chronic nociplastic pain that we see the greatest kinship between pain and suffering, between pain and other negative affective states like anxiety and depression. Understanding this kinship is crucial to providing better care for patients with these types of problems. For too long, we have distinguished pain as a physical state from suffering as a mental state. This is too facile and too dualistic. Pain has intrinsic emotional features, even if they are not universal. Pain after completing a marathon or delivering a baby can have joyous flavor. Suffering has intrinsic physical features, even if they are not universal. Not everyone with heartbreak will have chest pain, not everyone with stage fright will have butterflies in their stomach. Klein is right that not all pain produces suffering and that not all suffering produces pain. For philosophical purposes of keeping concepts crisp and clear, emphasizing these differences is fine. But for clinical purposes, it risks harming patients with over-medicalized pain treatments.

3.6 Pain, Anxiety, and Depression as Homeostatic Emotions

The subjective experience of pain is not equivalent to the objective neuronal activation of nociception. Pain is also not equivalent to suffering, anxiety, or depression. However, there is greater kinship among these states than is generally appreciated when we see pain as a mechanically generated response to injury and suffering as an emotional reaction to the sensation of pain. Neuroscientists Baliki and Apkarian can help us understand pain, anxiety, and depression all as protective homeostatic emotions.[24] "Pain and negative moods are envisioned as a continuum of aversive behavioral learning, which enhance survival by protecting against threats." These protect not only biological integrity, but in humans also protect personal and agential integrity. This latter form of integrity consists of the ability to be an agent in the world, to have relationships, and to accomplish goals.

Each step in the progression of nociception to pain to behavior is modulated by the brain to serve homeostasis. This begins with the translation of nociception into acute pain. Not all nociception is translated into conscious pain; much of it is silent. Currently the nociceptors in my buttocks and thighs are active as I sit writing this, but I shift my position in my chair before I feel pain. Similarly, I walk, run, and jump in ways that do not damage my joints, unlike persons with a congenital insensitivity to pain. Baliki and Apkarian explain, "As a result, the nociceptive control of behavior routinely occurs in the absence of consciously perceived pain, rendering it 'subconscious.'" This "protects the organism from tissue damage." Although the translation of nociception into pain is continuously modulated, the nociception-to-pain threshold is not fixed but adjusted by "cortical and limbic inputs that reflect past experiences, values, expectations, and salience relative to the self." This represents a "counterbalance between reward and aversion within the context of the learned history." Baliki and Apkarian modify Klein's claim about the protective function of pain: "Acute pain is not a warning signal but rather is the failure of the machinery (nociceptive activity) designed to avoid pain." In many cases, the experience of pain is not necessary to achieve tissue protection. Conscious pain functions, therefore, not to prevent initial damage, but to "protect the organism from further injury and promote healing." A significant portion of the cortical mantle (about 15%) is responsive to nociceptive stimuli. But, as reviewed in the preceding section on the salience network, this cortex also responds to non-nociceptive stimuli. It is also true that this cortical activity is not directly predictive of the perceived magnitude of pain.

Just as the translation of nociception into acute pain is modulated to maintain homeostasis, so also is the translation of acute pain into chronic pain. These are generally longer-term shifts in threshold mechanisms that are driven by limbic circuitry shaped by synaptic learning-based reorganization. Baliki and Apkarian explain how reward circuitry regulates pain perception: "Ventral striatal circuitry links nociception, acute pain, and chronic pain. This circuitry assesses salience for impending pain as well as expected reward value for relief of pain" (p. 482). In the only study to date that prospectively investigated the transition from acute to chronic low back pain, Hashmi, Baliki, Apkarian, and colleagues showed how, over the span of a year, brain activity associated with back pain on fMRI shifted away from sensory to emotional/limbic brain regions.[25] This occurs even though the study subjects with persistent back pain said that their experience of back pain was unchanged during this time. The persistence of back pain through the 1-year follow-up period was predicted best by corticostriatal functional connectivity between the nucleus accumbens and the prefrontal cortex.[26] Thus the strength of a reward circuit best predicted what is generally interpreted as the persistence of the sensory state of back pain.

These data can help us understand the relationships among chronic pain, anxiety, and depression. We have reviewed how pain motivates activity to avoid further injury and promote healing. We can extend this homeostatic model to understand anxiety as an emotional state characterized by sympathetic arousal that "promotes behaviors that diminish anticipated danger within one's immediate physical space and at relatively short time scales." This model can be extended further to include depression as "a more global generalization of perceived aversiveness of one's environment." Each of these homeostatic emotions protects the organism from immediate danger (pain), proximate danger (anxiety), and more distant and global danger (depression) by limiting behavior. Baliki explains, "structural and functional alterations in the ventral-tegmental striatal circuitry associated with anhedonia are consistent with the threshold phenomena we have discussed for pain" (p. 484). Chronic pain and depression are both associated with decreased volumes in the hippocampus and amygdala. These have also been reported in posttraumatic stress disorder (PTSD). These are conditions known to be common in patients with chronic pain and to worsen chronic pain outcomes. Now it appears that they share a neurobiological basis as well. "Overall, there seems to be a remarkable overlap between brain structures that either impart vulnerability or are affected by pain chronification and pathological negative moods."

The clinical advantages of viewing pain, anxiety, and depression as homeostatic emotions are many. Although many clinicians and patients with chronic pain embrace the acute pain model of an injury-induced sensory event inducing an emotional reaction, this is not adequate to direct care. It overemphasizes the peripheral and nociceptive features of chronic pain as causal.[27] It encourages searching for and repairing the broken body part in conditions like chronic back pain and fibromyalgia, where this search retards recovery and leads to iatrogenic injury.[28] It frames psychological and social interventions as addressing only the consequences of chronic pain and not its causes.[29]

If we instead frame chronic pain, anxiety, and depression as protective behavioral drives that inhibit exploratory, potentially risky, behavior, new conceptual and therapeutic options emerge. Depressive symptoms like anhedonia and social withdrawal are rightly seen as pathologies that inhibit recovery and prolong suffering. But these can also assist with disengaging from futile projects that only deplete personal resources.[30] Understanding that chronic pain, as well as anxiety and depression, are protective responses caused by a broad sense of danger rather than tissue damage opens up new therapeutic possibilities. Therapies that address and reduce this sense of danger can then be seen as addressing the causes of chronic pain and not simply its effects. These therapies can aim for the reduction or elimination of chronic pain rather than just improving coping or reducing disability. Therapies based on these ideas have shown promise in early trials. Pain neuroscience education (PNE) or the "explain pain" model developed by Moseley and colleagues in Australia has shown promise, especially when combined with other pain rehabilitation efforts.[31] Pain reprocessing therapy (PRT) has shown that it can reduce or eliminate back pain in community samples.[32] The PRT model has been supplemented with greater attention to trauma in the kind of chronic pain patients who are seen in pain clinics

32 MARK D. SULLIVAN

in emotional awareness and expression therapy (EAET). This therapy adds emotion induction and expressive writing exercises to the basic PRT model to extend its reach and has shown promise in preliminary trials.[33–35]

3.7 Opioids, Pain, and Depression

In the days before the opioid epidemic was launched, it was hoped by many that providing pain relief to injured workers would promote rehabilitation and return to work. By reducing pain with an early opioid prescription, movement and rehabilitation would become possible and lead to resumption of work. However, multiple prospective cohort studies have shown that this is not true.[36,37] The reasons for this failure are not entirely clear, but it appears that the deactivating effect of opioid therapy is more important than its analgesic effect, especially when that therapy is long-term.[38]

These effects of opioid medications can be explained by the interaction of continuous long-term opioid therapy with the endogenous opioid system. Exogenous opioid medications exert their multiple effects by interacting with the mu, kappa, and delta receptors of this endogenous system. It is very important to note that this system does not only continuously modulate pain to promote survival, as discussed above. The endogenous opioid system also regulates reward of all types, restores the organism after steroid-induced stress responses, and supports essential human social functions.[39] This system has been noted to be abnormal in both chronic pain and depression through functional neuroimaging studies.[40,41] Appropriate and efficient function of the endogenous opioid system depends on balancing the tonic and phasic release of opioids, which is likely disrupted by continuous exposure to opioid medications.

In pharmaco-epidemiological studies, depression is associated with increased opioid use.[42] Depression has small effects on rates of initial opioid prescribing, but at least doubles the likelihood of short-term opioid use advancing to long-term opioid use.[43] These increased rates of long-term use cannot be explained by better pain relief because multiple studies have shown that depressed patients with chronic pain get less pain relief from opioids than do non-depressed patients.[44] Long-term opioid use not only fails to relieve depression but is likely to induce it, especially with high-dose, continuous use.[45,46] Patients with significant psychological trauma and PTSD have high rates of long-term opioid use.[47] These opioid medications appear to provide some relief for the insomnia and hyperarousal aspects of PTSD but worsen the avoidance and withdrawal aspects of PTSD.[48]

Although explanations of legitimate opioid use usually refer to the production of pain relief and explanations of illicit opioid abuse refer to the production of euphoria, these may not best capture opioid effects. The feeling that opioids create, whether used licitly or illicitly, is best described as "safety." This is best evoked by opioid addicts interviewed by the *New York Times*, who explained that using heroin is "like being hugged by God." This feeling of perfect safety can be achieved through opioids even though one's life has fallen apart, one is living on the streets, and one is generally less safe than ever before. This pharmacologically induced sense of safety directly addresses the function of the homeostatic emotions of pain, anxiety, and depression that are behavioral drives aimed at preventing further injury. If we are to provide effective non-opioid treatments for chronic pain, they, too, will need to increase the patient's sense of safety with movement, social activity, and general adult responsibilities.

3.8 Conclusion

In our modern era, we separate pain from the rest of human suffering as a uniquely medical and mechanical experience. We feel comfortable calling on the medical system to provide relief of this pain, whether it be acute or chronic. The push for patients' right to pain relief is one of the deepest roots of the opioid epidemic. This is because the assertion of a right to pain relief assumes that pain relief can be delivered by medical professionals and that the patient has no role in producing that relief other than submitting to recommended medical treatment. We discuss this in more detail in our book, *The Right to Pain Relief and Other Deep Roots of the Opioid Epidemic*.[49]

As we further explore non-opioid treatments for chronic pain, we need to explore the relationship between pain and suffering without the assumption that pain is the cause and suffering is the effect. All pain has an affective component that is motivating. Some of this is intrinsic to pain and requires no cognition. Some pain affect is amplified by cognitions such as catastrophizing. Much of pain is associated with suffering. Suffering can also produce pain.

Eric Cassell famously defined suffering as "the state of severe distress associated with events that threaten the intactness of the person."[50]

34 MARK D. SULLIVAN

Cassell's concept of the "person" includes relationships, projects, goals, and obligations. We have traditionally understood pain as something that happens to the body and suffering as something that happens to the person. But this easy dualism is undercut by the view of pain as a homeostatic emotion that we have reviewed above. This view can help explain why an increased sense of safety can reduce not only pain unpleasantness, but also pain intensity. It helps us understand that, for humans, safety extends beyond bodily integrity to include personal integrity, which encompasses the same relationships, projects, goals, and obligations that Cassell considered part of personhood.

This draws attention to how pain can be an assault on our sense of self or personhood. It is not just a sensation followed by reflex withdrawal. Conscious pain allows for delay and flexibility in our response to a threat that is not possible with reflex withdrawal. It allows for the balancing of pain with other rewards and threats relevant to survival.[51] Humans are complex organisms whose safety depends not only on preserving themselves as a biological unity through homeostasis. Human safety depends on social agency and social integration.[52] When this agency is threatened by trauma or abuse, our personal integrity is endangered and chronic pain can result.

References

1. Price DD *Psychological and Neural Mechanisms of Pain.* Raven Press; 1988.
2. Sherrington C. *The Integrative Action of the Nervous System.* Constable; 1906.
3. Melzack R. The McGill Pain Questionnaire: Major properties and scoring methods. *Pain.* 1975;1(3):277–299.
4. Rainville P, Carrier B, Hofbauer RK, Bushnell MC, Duncan GH. Dissociation of sensory and affective dimensions of pain using hypnotic modulation. *Pain.* 1999;82(2):159–171.
5. Craig A. A new view of pain as a homeostatic emotion. *Trends Neurosci.* 2003;26(6):303–307.
6. Craig A. Pain mechanisms: Labeled lines versus convergence in central processing. *Annu Rev Neurosci* 2003;26:1–30.
7. Craig A. Cooling, pain, and other feelings from the body in relation to the autonomic nervous system. *Handb Clin Neurol.* 2013;117:103–109.
8. Klein C. *What the Body Commands: The Imperative Theory of Pain.* MIT Press; 2015.
9. Malterud K. Medically unexplained symptoms: Are we making progress? *Br J Gen Pract.* 2019;69(681):164–165.
10. Jackson JL, Kroenke K. Managing somatization: Medically unexplained should not mean medically ignored. *J Gen Intern Med.* 2006;21(7):797–799.
11. Rhodes LA, McPhillips-Tangum CA, Markham C, Klenk R. The power of the visible: The meaning of diagnostic tests in chronic back pain. *Soc Sci Med.* 1999;48(9):1189–1203.
12. Jensen MC, Brant-Zawadzki MN, Obuchowski N, Modic MT, Malkasian D, Ross JS. Magnetic resonance imaging of the lumbar spine in people without back pain. *N Engl J Med.* 1994;331(2):69–73.

13. Graves J, Fulton-Kehoe, D, Jarvik JG, Franklin GM. Early imaging for acute low back pain: one-year health and disability outcomes among Washington State workers. *Spine.* 2012;37(18):1617–1627.
14. Jacobs JC JJ, Chou R, Boothroyd D, Lo J, Nevedal A, Barnett PG. Observational study of the downstream consequences of inappropriate MRI of the lumbar spine. *J Gen Intern Med.* 2020;35(12):3605–3612.
15. Coghill RC, Sang CN, Maisog JM, Iadarola MJ. Pain intensity processing within the human brain: A bilateral, distributed mechanism. *J Neurophysiol* 1999;82:1934–1943.
16. Iannetti GD, Hughes NP, Lee MC, Mouraux A. Determinants of laserevoked EEG responses: Pain perception or stimulus saliency? *J Neurophysiol.* 2008;100:815–828.
17. Kucyi A, Davis KD. The neural code for pain: From single-cell electrophysiology to the dynamic pain connectome. *Neuroscientist.* 2017 Aug;23(4):397–414.
18. Borsook D, Edwards R, Elman I, Becerra L, Levine J. Pain and analgesia: The value of salience circuits. *Prog Neurobiol.* 2013;104:93–105.
19. Legrain V, Iannetti GD, Plaghki L, Mouraux A. The pain matrix reloaded: A salience detection system for the body. *Prog Neurobiol.* 2011;93(1):111–124.
20. Iannetti GD, Mouraux A. From the neuromatrix to the pain matrix (and back). *Exp Brain Res.* 2010;205(1):1–12.
21. Legrain V, Mancini F, Sambo CF, Torta DM, Ronga I, Valentini E. Cognitive aspects of nociception and pain: Bridging neurophysiology with cognitive psychology. *Neurophysiol Clin.* 2012;42(5):325–336.
22. Löwe B, Kroenke K, Spitzer RL, Williams JB, et al. Trauma exposure and posttraumatic stress disorder in primary care patients: Cross-sectional criterion standard study. *J Clin Psychiatry.* 2011;72(3):304–312.
23. Wall P. On the relation of injury to pain. The John J. Bonica lecture. *Pain.* 1979;6(3):253–264.
24. Baliki MN, Apkarian AV. Nociception, pain, negative moods, and behavior selection. *Neuron.* 2015;87(3):474–491.
25. Hashmi JA, Baliki MN, Huang L, et al. Shape shifting pain: Chronification of back pain shifts brain representation from nociceptive to emotional circuits. *Brain.* 2013;136(Pt 9):2751–2768.
26. Baliki M, Petre B, Torbey S, et al. Corticostriatal functional connectivity predicts transition to chronic back pain. *Nat Neurosci.* 2012;15(8):1117–1119.
27. Sullivan MD SJ, Lumley MA, Ballantyne JC. Reconsidering Fordyce's classic article, "Pain and suffering: what is the unit?" to help make our model of chronic pain truly biopsychosocial. *Pain.* 2023 Feb 1;164(2):271–279.
28. Cherkin DC, Deyo RA, Goldberg H. Time to align coverage with evidence for treatment of back pain. *J Gen Intern Med.* 2019;34(9):1910–1912.
29. Edwards RR, Dworkin RH, Sullivan MD, Turk DC, Wasan AD. The role of psychosocial processes in the development and maintenance of chronic pain. *J Pain.* 2016;17(9 Suppl):T70–92.
30. Nesse RM. Is depression an adaptation? *Arch Gen Psychiatry.* 2000;57(1):14–20.
31. Moseley GL, Butler DS. Fifteen years of explaining pain: The past, present, and future. *J Pain.* 2015;16(9):807–813.
32. Ashar Y, Gordon A, Schubiner H, et al. Effect of pain reprocessing therapy vs placebo and usual care for patients with chronic back pain: A randomized clinical trial. *JAMA Psychiatry.* 2022;79(1):13–23.
33. Lumley M, Schubiner H, Lockhart NA, et al. Emotional awareness and expression therapy, cognitive behavioral therapy, and education for fibromyalgia: A cluster-randomized controlled trial. *Pain.* 2017;158(12):2354–2363.
34. Lumley M, Schubiner H. Emotional awareness and expression therapy for chronic pain: Rationale, principles and techniques, evidence, and critical review. *Curr Rheumatol Rep.* 2019;21(7):30.

36 MARK D. SULLIVAN

35. Maroti D, Lumley MA, Schubiner H, et al. Internet-based emotional awareness and expression therapy for somatic symptom disorder: A randomized controlled trial. *J Psychosom Res.* 2022;163:111068.
36. Franklin GM, Stover BD, Turner JA, Fulton-Kehoe D, Wickizer TM, Disability Risk Identification Study C. Early opioid prescription and subsequent disability among workers with back injuries: The Disability Risk Identification Study Cohort. *Spine (Phila Pa 1976).* 2008;33(2):199–204.
37. Franklin GM, Fulton-Kehoe D, Turner JA, Wickizer T. Prescription opioid use and the risk of disability. *Clin J Pain.* 2018;34(2):190.
38. Ballantyne JC, Sullivan MD, Koob GF. Refractory dependence on opioid analgesics. *Pain.* 2019. Dec;160(12):2655–2660.
39. Ballantyne JC, Sullivan MD. The discovery of endogenous opioid systems: What it has meant for understanding pain and its treatment. *Pain.* 2017 Dec;158(12):2290–2300.
40. Light SN, Bieliauskas LA, Zubieta JK. "Top-down" mu-opioid system function in humans: Mu-opioid receptors in ventrolateral prefrontal cortex mediate the relationship between hedonic tone and executive function in major depressive disorder. *J Neuropsychiatry Clin Neurosci.* 2017 Fall;29(4):357–364.
41. Kennedy SE, Koeppe RA, Young EA, Zubieta JK. Dysregulation of endogenous opioid emotion regulation circuitry in major depression in women. *Arch Gen Psychiatry.* 2006;63(11):1199–1208.
42. Sullivan MD. Depression effects on long-term prescription opioid use, abuse, and addiction. *Clin J Pain.* 2018;34(9):878–884.
43. Sullivan MD. Commentary on Higgins et al. (2020): How are chronic pain, psychological distress and opioid dependence related? *Addiction.* 2020;115(2):259–260.
44. Wasan AD, Michna E, Edwards RR, et al. Psychiatric comorbidity is associated prospectively with diminished opioid analgesia and increased opioid misuse in patients with chronic low back pain. *Anesthesiology.* 2015;123(4):861–872.
45. Scherrer JF, Salas J, Sullivan MD, et al. The influence of prescription opioid use duration and dose on development of treatment resistant depression. *Prev Med.* 2016;91:110–116.
46. Scherrer JF, Salas J, Copeland LA, et al. Prescription opioid duration, dose, and increased risk of depression in 3 large patient populations. *Ann Fam Med.* 2016;14(1):54–62.
47. Elman I, Borsook D. The failing cascade: Comorbid post traumatic stress- and opioid use disorders. *Neurosci Biobehav Rev.* 2019;103:374–383.
48. Smith KZ, Smith PH, Cercone SA, McKee SA, Homish GG. Past year non-medical opioid use and abuse and PTSD diagnosis: Interactions with sex and associations with symptom clusters. *Addict Behav.* 2016;58:167–174.
49. Sullivan M, Ballantyne JC. *The Right to Pain Relief and Other Deep Roots of Our Opioid Epidemic.* Oxford University Press; 2023.
50. Cassell E. *The Nature of Suffering and the Goals of Medicine.* 2nd ed. Oxford University Press; 2004.
51. Fuchs T. *Ecology of the Brain.* Oxford University Press; 2018.
52. Wilson EO. *The Social Conquest of Earth.* Norton; 2012.

4

Prescription Opioid Use and Risk of Depression and Worsening Mental Health

Jeffrey F. Scherrer and Joanne Salas

4.1 Overview

Numerous studies demonstrate that persons with prescription opioid misuse, non-medical opioid use, and opioid use disorder have an increased risk for a variety of psychiatric disorders, particularly depression.[1-3] A separate body of research indicates that the risk for depression is elevated among patients who use prescription opioids for non-cancer pain, and this risk for depression is independent of opioid use disorder.[4,5] Thus, patients who take opioids as prescribed for non-cancer pain may unintentionally be increasing risk for new-onset or worsening depression. Because many patients attribute depression to pain, determining if opioids are associated with increased depression risk informs pain management and safe opioid prescribing as well as provides insights into the role of the endogenous opioid system in mood disorders. This chapter is focused on developing the evidence for an association between long-term prescription opioid use for non-cancer pain and risk for new-onset depression and worsening depression.

The body of work on the relationship between prescription opioid use and risk for developing depression comes from a variety of study designs including retrospective cohort studies that use de-identified data from electronic health records, prospective cohort studies, and cross-sectional data. While others have shown that non-medical opioid use and opioid misuse are risk factors for depression and other mood disorders,[1] this chapter is focused on studies measuring duration and dose of prescription opioid use and risk for new-onset and worsening depression.

Jeffrey F. Scherrer and Joanne Salas, *Prescription Opioid Use and Risk of Depression and Worsening Mental Health*
In: *Pain, the Opioid Epidemic, & Depression*. Edited by: Jeffrey F. Scherrer & Jane C. Ballantyne, Oxford University Press.
© Oxford University Press 2024. DOI: 10.1093/9780197675250.003.0004

38 JEFFREY F. SCHERRER AND JOANNE SALAS

No randomized clinical trials are designed to determine whether prescription opioid use leads to new-onset or worsening depression. It would be unethical to randomize patients to a potentially harmful dose or duration of opioid analgesics; therefore, most research in this area has relied on cohort designs. These include prospective and retrospective cohorts. The latter typically uses de-identified medical claims or medical record data which contain diagnoses and information about opioid prescriptions.

We begin this chapter by first defining key constructs in this field. Because this chapter reports the findings from a series of studies employing complex analyses of historical, de-identified medical records and medical claims, we discuss details important to understanding the retrospective cohort design. But first, to understand the extant literature on prescription opioid use and depression, the approach to measuring non-cancer pain, prescription opioid characteristics, and depression all need to be described. Variation in how these variables are measured might explain some of the inconsistencies in the literature.

4.2 Measuring Non-Cancer Pain

Acute pain is short-lived and may follow surgery, a fall, or other injuries. According to the International Association for the Study of Pain,[6] "Acute pain happens suddenly, starts out sharp or intense, and serves as a warning sign of disease or threat to the body. It is caused by injury, surgery, illness, trauma, or painful medical procedures and generally lasts from a few minutes to less than six months. Acute pain usually disappears whenever the underlying cause is treated or healed."[6]

Acute pain may transition to *chronic pain*, the latter defined as pain on most days lasting more than 3 months.[7] Factors contributing to this transition include comorbid psychiatric disorders, smoking, and pain-related impaired functioning.[8] Non-cancer chronic pain may continue long after the inciting process has resolved. Some studies of prescription opioid use and risk for depression are focused on patients with chronic non-cancer pain,[9,10] and others have defined pain as any non-cancer pain condition for which an opioid may be prescribed.[4,11] Because opioids may be prescribed for both acute and chronic pain, measuring the association between prescription opioid use and new-onset depression requires disentangling the associations between pain, opioid use, and depression.

4.3 Defining Long-Term Opioid Therapy

A new period of opioid use is defined as starting a prescription opioid after 6 or more months without opioid use. This definition has been adopted in numerous opioid pharmaco-epidemiological studies.[12-14] *Chronic opioid use* or *long-term opioid therapy* (LTOT) has typically been defined as using a prescription opioid for 90 days or longer.

Opioids studied include immediate and extended-release formulations for codeine, dihydrocodeine, fentanyl, hydrocodone, hydromorphone, levorphanol, meperidine, methadone, morphine, oxycodone, oxymorphone, pentazocine, tapentadol, and tramadol. In studies using data prior to 2012, it was uncommon to see substantial tramadol prescribing. In addition, buprenorphine was not included in opioid exposures because it was difficult to determine when it was prescribed for pain versus prescribed for opioid use disorder.

To compute opioid use duration, most studies begin by measuring the date of medication fill for any prescription opioid at any dose. In retrospective cohort studies using medical record data, it is common to measure the duration of opioid use with the "days supply" measure, accounting for overlapping fills/days. Days supply is the amount of time it would take for the patient to use all of their medication if taken as prescribed and is used to calculate an end date per fill. Patients are considered continuous users until a gap of greater than 30 days occurs since their last fill. At that point, the duration of the new period of opioid use is considered to have ended. The duration of that continuous use period is the difference between the end date of the last fill and start date of the first fill in that period. In this example, LTOT includes a mix of daily, frequent, and intermittent use. In other prospective and retrospective studies, long-term opioid use has been defined according to the Consortium to Study Opioid Risks and Trends (CONSORT) definition. CONSORT defines LTOT as a period of opioid use of 90 days during which the patient had 120 days supply or greater or 10 or more opioid prescriptions dispensed within a given year.[15,16]

Some patients receive two types of opioids, one for regular use and one for breakthrough pain. This overlap is usually not counted twice when computing the total opioid use duration. For instance, a patient who has 3 months of a prescription opioid dispensed and has a 7-day supply of another opioid for breakthrough pain would be counted as having 3 months of opioid use. Differences in the definitions used to measure LTOT and frequency of opioid

40 JEFFREY F. SCHERRER AND JOANNE SALAS

use among patients with non-cancer pain may explain some of the inconsistent evidence regarding LTOT and new-onset depression.

4.4 Considerations for Standardizing Dosage

Each prescription opioid contains a different amount of morphine per 1 mg of medication. Therefore, to measure opioid dose, it is necessary to standardize the dose of individual opioid medications to the morphine milligram equivalent (MME) dose. The MME is computed from widely available conversion tables.[17] For example, 1 mg of hydrocodone converts to 1 mg of morphine, 1 mg of codeine equates to 0.1 mg morphine, and 1 mg oxycodone equals 1.5 mg morphine. When measuring daily dose using medical records or medical claims, it is common to assume patients use the maximum prescribed dose per day. Thus, daily dose is calculated as unit dose multiplied by quantity per day (i.e., total dispensed/days supply). Once the daily MME is obtained, several options are available for creating the dose exposure. Opioid dose has been measured as the average daily dose, maximum daily dose reached, change in dose over time, and total MME used over a specified period. While we lack robust evidence that higher MME is an independent risk factor for new-onset depression, more rapid dose escalation, compared to stable or decreasing dose, appears to increase risk for depression.[14] Rapid dose escalation may be a proxy for uncontrolled pain, problems with managing opioid use, and opioid misuse. These factors could all be associated with increased risk for depression. As discussed below, variation in how dose is modeled may explain different findings regarding high-dose opioid use and new-onset depression.

4.5 Pain as a Key Confounding Factor

To understand if LTOT is associated with an increased risk for new-onset depression, studies must implement robust control for bias by indication. As illustrated in Figure 4.1, bias by indication means that the reason for the treatment biases the measure of association between the treatment and the outcome. In the case of opioid use and risk for new-onset depression, bias by indication is present because patients are prescribed opioids for pain and pain is strongly correlated with depression.[18,19]

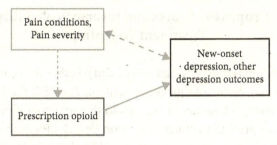

Figure 4.1 Bias by indication. Prescription opioids are indicated for pain and pain is associated with increased risk for depression.

Over the past few decades, a substantial literature has grown and consistently supports the link between pain and depression.[18,19] Patients with versus without depression are much more likely to develop pain conditions. Kroenke and colleagues[18] demonstrated a strong bidirectional relationship in that worsening pain leads to increases in depression symptoms, and, as pain decreases, so does depression severity. Patients with chronic pain who develop long-term opioid use may ascribe their comorbid depression to their pain condition.[20,21] While certainly pain interference and pain severity are associated with poor mood and more depression symptoms, growing evidence indicates that long-term opioid use can lead to new-onset depression independent of the relationship between pain and depression.

4.5.1 Controlling for Bias by Indication and Other Confounding

It would not be ethical to randomize patients to different opioid exposure levels, including levels that may increase risk for adverse outcomes. However, using quasi-experimental approaches with a large sample size, it is possible to remove meaningful differences in the distribution of pain conditions and pain severity across levels of opioid exposure. Removing such differences using statistical methods creates two or more groups who appear to have been randomized to an exposure. For example, the distribution of confounding factors would no longer differ between patients exposed to 1–30, 30–90, or more than 90 days of prescription opioid use. To accomplish balance, several methods are available, including the use of propensity scores (PS).

4.6 Propensity Scores and Inverse Probability of Treatment Weighting

Whether a patient is prescribed an opioid and whether they continue to use opioids for a long period of time is not random. The PS is the probability of a patient receiving a treatment (e.g., opioid therapy) conditional on measured covariates prior to treatment initiation.[22,23] The PS must only include baseline measures and not measures that could be impacted by the exposure. For example, pain severity measured up to the start of an opioid would be used in computing the PS but not pain severity after opioid initiation.[22] The PS is computed from a binary or multinomial logistic regression model that predicts the probability or propensity to receive a treatment, such as different durations of opioid therapy. The PS can also be computed using generalized boosted modeling, which is a more robust method than traditional regression modeling, especially in the case of multiple exposure groups. The PS can be used to match patient characteristics across different levels of opioid exposure. The PS can also be used to weight the data. By applying the PS and inverse probability of treatment weighting, balance across opioid exposure groups can be obtained. Weighting data using the PS creates a synthetic database and is similar to weights applied to survey sampling used to create a sample representative of the source population.[22] Weighting or matching on the PS is a critical step in measuring real-world outcomes in cohorts assigned to a treatment based on their exposures to opioid therapy as measured in the medical record. Successful matching or weighting results in balancing the distribution of confounding factors between opioid exposures such that there are no meaningful differences between those who do or do not receive an opioid. Weighting can also be used to balance the distribution of potential confounding variables across multiple groups, such as those with 1- to 30-day, 31- to 90-day, and more than 90-day opioid use. A common effect size measure, *standardized mean difference*, assesses covariate balance, and a threshold of less than 0.10 is commonly used to conclude balance has been achieved (i.e., no meaningful difference exists in the distribution of confounders between exposure groups).[22]

Using the PS to compute stabilized, inverse probability of treatment weights (IPTW) and then weighting the data retains the original number of patients. Weighting is sometimes preferred over matching on the PS because the latter approach will lead to lost sample size because it is not always possible to match all subjects. Weighted data are then used to generate an unbiased association between opioid use and new-onset depression. Randomizing is intended to remove differences between treated and untreated patients. Similarly, using PS and IPTW, patients who have greater than 90 days opioid exposure versus less than 90 days opioid exposure, or those with versus without an opioid prescription, will not differ, on average, in the distribution of confounding factors and covariates.[22] Figure 4.2 gives an example of covariate distributions, computed from fabricated data, before and after weighting.

Computing the association between opioid duration and new-onset depression in weighted data permits estimating the total effect of opioid duration and risk for new-onset depression, independent of pain, nicotine dependence, anxiety disorders, pain conditions, etc. This method was

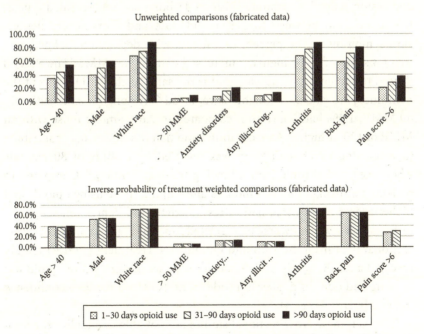

Figure 4.2 Distribution of potential confounding variables before and after weighting.

applied in numerous retrospective cohort studies testing the association between duration of opioid use and new-onset depression,[4] transition from depression to treatment-resistant depression,[24] and frequency of opioid use in LTOT and new-onset depression,[13] as well as in investigation of opioid use and risk of depression recurrence.[25]

4.7 Summary of Evidence from Existing Cross-Sectional Studies

Before discussing the larger body of evidence from retrospective and prospective cohort studies, it should be noted that the first evidence for a link between prescription opioid use and depression surfaced with several cross-sectional studies.

The first report of an association between prescription opioid use and depression was a cross-sectional survey of chronic prescription opioid users who completed the Patient Health Questionnaire 8-item (PHQ-8) depression scale.[26] A separate study of 43 burn patients revealed a positive association between higher opioid dose and more severe depression symptoms.[27] The percent of patients with depression, defined as a PHQ-8 score of 10 or higher,[28] increased with higher MME. The PHQ-8 is used to screen for depression and is the same as the PHQ-9 except the item querying suicidal thoughts is removed.[28] Among patients with 20–49 MME, 1.4% had depression compared to 2.6% among those with an MME of 120 or higher. An early indication that opioid use may contribute to worsening psychopathology was revealed by a study of 80 patients who developed chronic pain following traumatic injury.[29] Compared to patients not using opioids 4 months after injury, those using opioids had higher scores on posttraumatic stress, anxiety, and depression screening instruments as well as worse pain-related functioning.[29] Analyses of cross-sectional data from the Pain and Opioids IN Treatment (POINT) study revealed a small, nearly null, association between duration of opioid use in years and odds of depression (odds ratio [OR] = 1.03; 95% confidence interval [CI]: 1.01, 1.04).[10]

However, these cross-sectional studies are not able to establish the temporal order of opioid use and depression. It could be that those with psychopathology had greater pain sensitivity or pain catastrophizing or self-medicated with opioids. Thus, underlying mental illness—including depression symptoms—could have led to requiring higher doses for pain relief or remaining on opioids for a longer period of time.

4.8 Results from Existing Retrospective Cohort Studies: Risks for New-Onset Depression

Since 1999, the Veterans Health Administration (VHA) has maintained a nationally distributed database of administrative medical records. These de-identified medical record data contain discrete fields in the electronic health record such as International Classification of Diseases (ICD) diagnoses codes (ICD-9 and ICD-10); Current Procedural Terminology (CPT) codes; prescriptions dispensed including medication type, dose, and days supply; vital signs; vital status; clinic type; some patient-reported outcomes such as the PHQ-9; and modest demographic data including age, race, gender, and marital status. Similar administrative medical record data bases have been developed across the United States and in other countries. An excellent example of cohorts from private-sector healthcare systems includes the Health Care System Research Network (HCSRN) sites such as Henry Ford Health system and Kaiser Permanente. Replicating results in multiple patient samples from different healthcare systems increases confidence in findings, particularly when cohorts differ in terms of patient demographic and/or clinical characteristics.

4.8.1 Strengths and Weaknesses of Retrospective Cohort Studies

To judge the quality of evidence for an association between opioid use and risk for depression, it is important to understand the key strengths and limitations of the retrospective cohort study design. Understanding this design is critical because 11 out of the 16 studies designed to determine if prescription opioid use is associated with risk for depression use retrospective cohorts.

Many prospective cohort studies and almost all randomized clinical trials exclude patients who have severe illness and those who may be vulnerable to suicide or have complex, comorbid psychiatric conditions. Because patients do not actively participate in retrospective designs, these patients are not excluded. Prospective cohort studies require recruiting eligible patients and collecting data at specific intervals over many months or years. Due to mistrust of the medical system and past violations of human rights in medical research, it can be difficult to recruit a representative proportion of minorities and underserved persons. This is not a limitation in retrospective studies.

Studies using medical record data have been criticized for the sometimes uncertain accuracy of ICD-9 and ICD-10 diagnoses. However, for many key variables including depression, diagnostic algorithms have been developed with good to excellent agreement with gold standard measures. Although a single diagnosis for depression has poor agreement with medical chart abstraction,[30,31] requiring two depression diagnoses on separate visits in the same 12-month period or one inpatient discharge diagnosis for depression has excellent agreement with manual chart abstraction and self-report.[30,31] In some instances, diagnostic algorithms can prove as accurate as diagnostic interviews. Using two diagnostic codes for posttraumatic stress disorder (PTSD) within the same 4 months has an 82% positive predictive value when compared to a gold standard PTSD Checklist (PCL) score of 50 or greater,[32] and presence of two diagnostic codes has an 88.4% agreement with the Structured Clinical Interview for DSM-IV (SCID) lifetime PTSD diagnosis.[33] This is better or on par with diagnoses obtained from the World Health Organization Composite International Diagnostic Interview compared to a gold standard SCID diagnosis.[34,35]

A second potential limitation of the retrospective cohort design is the risk for unmeasured confounding. This means that an important confounder was either not included in the analyses or was not available in the medical record. For example, measures of social support, patient beliefs, and similar constructs do not exist in medical record data. However, these unmeasured confounding factors are often correlated with measured ones. The *e-value* has been proposed as a means to evaluate the potential impact of unmeasured confounding.[36] Two e-values can be computed, one for the point estimate and one for the CI of an estimated treatment effect. The point estimate e-value is the minimum association (e.g., minimum risk ratio, hazard ratio, OR, etc.) an unmeasured confounder would need with both the exposure and outcome to make the outcome effect estimate null. Similarly, the e-value

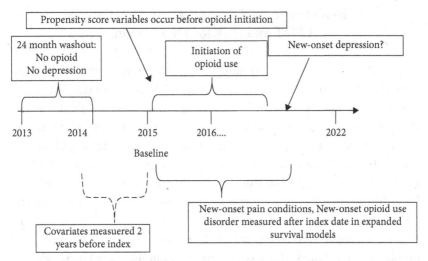

Figure 4.3 Retrospective cohort design.

for the CI is the minimum association needed with both the outcome and exposure to have the CI contain the null.

The majority of retrospective studies in this field have employed a "new user" design to measure the association between opioid use and new-onset depression or worsening depression. For opioid medications, this means that patients are eligible for the study if they have 6 months or longer without a prescribed opioid. Patients who receive opioids after 6 months without a prescription opioid are considered to be starting a new period of use. This does not mean patients have never been prescribed an opioid. Most patients with chronic pain are middle-aged, and there are few if any cohorts with decades of observation time to determine if middle-aged adults received opioids as adolescents or young adults. Therefore, in the new user design, the goal is to select patients without prevalent prescription opioid use to accurately measure the duration of a new prescription opioid episode. To measure new-onset depression, patients must have visits in the 2 years prior to opioid initiation and be free of any depression diagnoses (see Figure 4.3). Therefore, eligible subjects are users of the healthcare system who are free of depression for 2 years and have no opioid use for at least 6 months at baseline (i.e., index date). Cox proportional hazard models are computed to estimate the association between opioid exposure and new-onset depression, worsening depression, or depression recurrence.

4.9 Evidence from Retrospective Cohort Studies: LTOT and Risk for Depression

The first retrospective cohort study on this topic was done using a cohort created from U.S. VHA de-identified medical record databases. The cohort was originally designed to study depression and incident myocardial infarction.[5] Compared to VHA patients with 1–89 days of opioid use, those with 90–180 days of opioid use had a 24%, and those with greater than 180 days had a 51% greater risk for new-onset depression. Because the cohort was designed to study heart disease outcomes, this study was biased because patients were free of heart disease at baseline. Scherrer and colleagues,[37] using a cohort designed for studies of opioid use and new-onset depression, observed that, among VHA patients who used opioids for 1–30 days, those who remained opioid users for 31–90 days (hazard ratio [HR] = 1.18; 95% CI: 1.10, 1.25) and for more than 90 days (HR = 1.35; 95% CI:1.26, 1.44) had significantly increased risk for new-onset depression. This study used PS and IPTW to control confounding. The association between longer duration of opioid use and new-onset depression was independent of pain and other confounding factors, including maximum MME, measured prior to index date. Results remained stable after expanding survival models to account for pain that could occur after opioid initiation. These results were replicated in two private-sector healthcare systems. In fact, the magnitude of association between greater than 90-day opioid use and new-onset depression was larger in private-sector healthcare system patients as compared to VHA patients. In all three cohorts, there was no relationship between higher MME and new-onset depression after controlling for the same set of confounding factors plus controlling for duration of opioid use.

Two key conclusions can be made from these studies. First, a dose-response relationship exists between duration of opioid use and risk for depression. Second, VHA results were replicated in the two private-sector samples despite VHA patients having many more comorbidities and generally lower socioeconomic status (SES). The ability to replicate results in patient populations with quite different characteristics increases confidence in the evidence that longer duration of prescription opioid use is associated with increased risk for new-onset depression.

Additional studies in this VHA population were done to investigate whether prescription opioid use was associated with transitioning from depression to treatment-resistant depression[24] and recurrence of a depressive episode.[38] Using PS and weighting to control for confounding, in a sample of more than 6,000 VHA patients 18–80 years of age, those who received 31–90 days and more than 90 days of prescription opioids, compared to 1–30 days, had a 25% and 52% increased likelihood of transitioning from depression to treatment-resistant depression, respectively.[24] MME dose was not associated with treatment-resistant depression. Separately, after controlling for confounding, VHA patients who were in remission and then exposed to prescription opioids for non-cancer pain, compared to remaining without an opioid, had nearly a twofold increased risk for a recurring depressive episode.[25] Based on this body of work, the evidence suggests that prescription opioid use and duration of use, but not MME dose, contributes to new-onset depression, worsening depression, and depression recurrence. Subsequent analyses demonstrated that the risk for depression in long-term opioid use was similar in males and females.[39] Of note, all studies used PS and IPTW methods to control confounding, therefore the observed opioid–depression associations were independent of numerous risk factors for depression that are also correlated with opioid use, including pain.

To our knowledge there is only one other retrospective cohort study that has measured the association between prescription opioid use and risk for depression. Wilson and colleagues[40] analyzed private-sector medical claim data from 106,260 patients who underwent total knee or hip arthroplasty to determine if chronic opioid use was associated with new depression diagnoses. Long-term opioid use was defined according to the CONSORT definition presented earlier in this chapter.[16] Patients with only postoperative chronic opioid use had the largest odds of developing depression, followed by pre- and postoperative opioid use. Furthermore, patients who were only prescribed an opioid prior to surgery also had an increased risk for depression (OR = 1.88; 95% CI: 1.47, 2.40).[40]

4.10 Results from Prospective Cohort Studies

Prospective cohort studies enroll eligible patients and collect data prospectively, typically with repeated assessments obtained, most often, over fixed time intervals. For instance, enrolling patients who started a new opioid prescription and collecting data about depression at 6-month and 12-month follow-ups would be a prospective cohort study design that would allow measuring the relationship between a new period of opioid use and subsequent depression.

50 JEFFREY F. SCHERRER AND JOANNE SALAS

A prospective cohort study in primary care followed patients with non-cancer pain over a 2-year period and measured prescription opioid dose and depression symptoms.[41] Within-person analyses revealed that increasing MME from 0 to more than 50 MME was associated with nearly a 2.7 times greater odds of developing depression (measured with the PHQ-2) in follow-up. There was no association between increasing from 0 MME to 1–50 MME.[41] While this result appears to contradict evidence from retrospective cohort studies, duration of opioid use was not measured. It is possible that patients who increased dose to greater than 50 MME were also the longest-term opioid users. If this was the case, then results are consistent with retrospective cohort studies.

In a prospective cohort study of adults 45 years of age and older, Von Korff and colleagues[9] categorized opioid use into minimal/no use, intermittent/lower dose, and regular/higher dose use. They did not observe a significant association between opioid use category and depression (measured with the PHQ-8) at 4-month and 12-month follow-ups.[9] As the authors noted, the overall modest dose (50 MME) in regular users and the fact that only 22% of patients were regular, high-dose users could account for the lack of association. It is possible that intermittent opioid use is not sufficient to increase the risk for depression. Further evidence supporting this conclusion is discussed in Section 4.11.

Analyses of data from the Australian Pain and Opioids IN Treatment (POINT) study revealed that, compared to patients who developed depression prior to opioid use and those who never had depression, patients who developed depression after opioid initiation started opioids at an earlier age, used them for a longer period of time, had higher MME dose, had more severe prescription opioid difficulties, experienced more side effects, and were more likely to have social phobia.[10] However, after controlling for covariates, duration of opioid use was not significantly associated with new-onset depression.[10] While this study may seem to contradict results from retrospective cohort studies, it should be noted that the depression measures were categorized into "odds of depression after opioid use compared to no history of depression" and "odds of experiencing depression following opioid use as compared to depression prior to opioid use." Thus, direct comparison to the body of retrospective studies is constrained. Another explanation for the discrepancy between this prospective study and the body of literature from retrospective cohort designs is the possibility that the latter includes patients

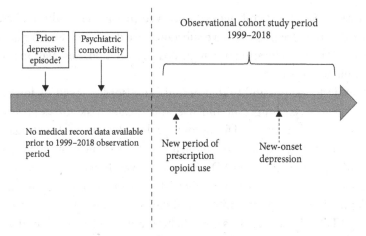

Figure 4.4 Factors preceding prescription opioid use may increase risk for incident mood disorder.

with a lifetime history of depression. As illustrated in Figure 4.4, the risk for depression following LTOT may be greatest or even limited to patients with a past history of depression.

4.11 Escalating Dose and Frequency of Use May Explain Risk for New-Onset Depression

Dose and duration are highly correlated. Longer-term prescription opioid users are more likely to be on higher doses than are short-term users.[4] Although maximum dose has not been found to be associated with risk for new-onset depression[42] changes in dose could be related to worsening mood and increased depression risk. Salas et al.[14] computed monthly dose trajectories in a cohort of 7,051 long-term (>90 day) opioid users. Stable, decreasing, slow increasing, and rapid increasing dose trajectories were identified. High MME was observed in the rapid increasers, with nearly 30% receiving more than 101 MME per day and 15% prescribed more than 180 MME per day. Interestingly, independent of the maximum dose and total duration of use, both slow increasers (HR = 1.22; 95% CI: 1.05, 1.42) and rapid increasers (HR = 1.58; 95% CI: 1.30, 1.93) had a significantly greater risk for new-onset depression compared to those receiving a stable dose. Why would MME dose escalation be associated with new-onset depression? Salas and colleagues[14] observed that patients who had a dose increase were more likely to have substance use disorders, which raises the question: Are long-duration use, high-dose use, and dose escalation proxies for opioid use disorder?

To exclude the possibility that opioid use disorder accounts for the association between longer opioid use and greater risk for depression, a subsequent study controlled for opioid use disorder when estimating the association between frequency of opioid use and risk for new-onset depression in a sample of patients with LTOT. This study was designed to overcome the limitation in prior retrospective cohort studies which did not separate risk for depression among intermittent and daily or near-daily opioid users receiving LTOT. To address this issue, Scherrer and colleagues[13] used a commercial, private-sector database of nationally distributed medical records integrated with medical claims to create a cohort of patients with 90 days of opioid use. Patients were then categorized into frequency of use in the initial 90-day opioid use period. The following groups were defined: (1) patients who had less than 50% days out of the first 90 days of opioid use covered (in other words, they had enough pills to use an opioid less than 45 out of 90 days); (2) intermittent users who had 45–71 days covered; (3) frequent users who had 72–80 days covered; and (4) daily users who had more than 80 days covered. After controlling for confounding using PS and IPTW, frequent (HR = 1.29; 95% CI: 1.01, 1.64) and daily users (HR = 1.32; 95% CI: 1.07, 1.63), compared to occasional users, had a significantly increased risk for new-onset depression even after controlling for pain conditions that could onset after opioid initiation. Most importantly, results were nearly identical after controlling for opioid use disorder following the first 90 days of opioid use. This refines our understanding of long-term opioid use and new-onset depression. Those most at risk for new-onset depression are long-term (i.e., >90 days) frequent or daily users, and this is not explained by whether a patient develops opioid use disorder. Daily or near-daily prescription opioid use may impair the endogenous opioid system and lead to poor hedonic tone.[43] This would reduce patients' ability to experience pleasure from naturally rewarding stimuli. These patients may also be more likely to develop hyperkatifeia. *Hyperkatifeia* is a negative emotional state involving malaise, irritability, unease, dysphoria, alexithymia, and anxiety.[44] This negative reinforcement may contribute to prescription opioid use disorder, to the degree that patients with LTOT use opioids to avoid these negative symptoms.[43,44]

4.12 Is Depression a Side Effect or Consequence of Long-Term Opioid Use?

Prescription opioids have side effects that overlap with some symptoms of depression. These include difficulty concentrating, fatigue, and lack of motivation or interest. Therefore, new-onset depression may be a side effect of prescription opioid use. We are aware of only one analysis that measured the time between LTOT and onset of depression. Among VHA patients who developed new-onset depression after 1–30, 31–90, and more than 90 days of opioid use, 93.2% of new depression cases occurred after the period of opioid use ended.[37] Among these patients, 82.9% were diagnosed with depression 6 months after opioid use stopped. The average duration from the end of a new period of opioid use and onset of depression was 3.4 years (standard deviation [SD] = 2.5 years).[4] This supports the conclusion that depression is a consequence of long-term opioid use and not a side effect. However, caution is warranted because there are delays between the time a patient develops symptoms of depression and when a diagnosis is obtained. Nonetheless, depression as a consequence of LTOT is consistent with evidence, expanded upon in Section 4.15, that opioid-related changes in reward centers in the brain remain long after opioid use stops.

4.13 Does Opioid Use Lead Specifically to Major Depressive Episodes or to Psychopathology in General?

The studies discussed in this chapter have all used either a screening instrument for depression such as the PHQ-9 or ICD-9 and ICD-10 codes to define depression. ICD-9 and ICD-10 codes may not always meet the criteria of the latest *Diagnostic and Statistical Manual of Mental Disorders* (DSM-5) for a major depressive episode. For example, patients diagnosed with depression may really have dysthymia or some other mood disturbance. More frequent illicit opioid use can lead to anhedonia independent of depression and PTSD.[45] Garland and colleagues[46] observed elevated anhedonia in patients with chronic pain, but only opioid misuse—not opioid use duration, dose, or pain severity—was associated with higher levels of anhedonia.

Trevino et al.[29] followed 101 trauma patients for 4 months and observed evidence for a higher prevalence of depression and anxiety symptoms among those who remained on opioids versus those who did not. However,

54 JEFFREY F. SCHERRER AND JOANNE SALAS

the small sample size reduced the ability to control a number of important confounding factors. Nonetheless, this study offers some evidence that long-term opioid use is associated with other psychiatric conditions and not just depression.

4.14 Does Long-Term Prescription Opioid Use Cause Depression?

Establishing evidence for causation is critical to developing effective interventions to prevent depression in patients who become chronic opioid users. To evaluate this question, we rely on the Bradford Hill criteria for causation.[47] The Hill criteria are strength of association, consistency, temporality, biological gradient/dose-response, biological plausibility, coherence, experimental evidence, and analogy. We have observed up to a two fold increased risk for depression in greater than 90-day opioid, users which is a strong association in retrospective cohort studies. All designs have established temporality in that prescription opioid use precedes new-onset depression. The biologic gradient or dose response criteria is met with evidence that greater than 90-day use is associated with a larger magnitude of risk for new-onset depression compared to 1–30 days and 31–89 days of use.[37] Biological plausibility is discussed below. Coherence is supported because the etiology of depression is consistent with the effects of opioids on mood. Last, analogy is present in that other mood disturbances, such as anhedonia and anxiety, are associated with LTOT.[29,46] Thus, most criteria for causation are met, but not all. Therefore, we are unable to conclude that prescription opioids or LTOT cause *incident* depression. It is possible that patients with past depressive episodes may be more likely to develop depression following opioid use. Persons with symptoms of depression, but insufficient to warrant a diagnosis, could experience worsening depression during or following LTOT that in turn leads to a depression diagnosis.

The most robust evidence for a causal relationship between opioid use and risk for depression is from a study using Mendelian randomization techniques. These methods use known genetic variants associated with a phenotype as proxies for the exposure under study.[48] The genetic variants serve as an *instrumental variable* that is associated with the exposure, is independent of confounders of the association between exposure and outcome, and the genetic variant contributes to the outcome via the exposure.[48] Using Mendelian randomization and data from genome-wide association studies, Rosoff and colleagues[49] observed the genetic liability for greater prescription opioid use was associated with liability for depression as well as for anxiety and stress-related disorders. Importantly, there was no association between nonopioid analgesics and depression or stress and anxiety. While this supports evidence for causation, the Mendelian randomization approach does not directly measure depression or prescription opioid use, and it is premature to conclude whether or not prescription opioid use causes depression.

4.15 Potential Biological Mechanisms

LTOT is associated with sleep disorders, including sleep apnea and impaired sleep.[50,51] Patients with sleep disorders, including insomnia, have a twofold increased risk for incident depression.[52] Thus, it is possible that LTOT could lead to sleep disorders, which in turn contribute to new-onset depression. Salas and colleagues[53] observed a trend for a stronger association between LTOT and new-onset depression among patients with versus without insomnia. Yet more frequent opioid use among LTOT remained associated with new-onset depression after controlling for sleep apnea.[13] Additional research is needed to clarify the role sleep may have in the opioid–depression relationship.

LTOT is a risk factor for hyperalgesia, an increased sensitivity to painful stimuli.[54] Therefore, patients may experience hyperalgesia following LTOT, which may contribute to worsening mood and risk for depression. We are not aware of studies that have investigated this pathway, but the strong evidence for a bidirectional relationship between more severe pain and increasing depression severity[18] supports this theory.

Biological mechanisms could also involve opioid-induced androgen deficiency. About 75% of patients on LTOT develop androgen deficiency, and one study observed 90% of cancer survivors receiving opioid treatment were hypogonadal.[55] Higher doses are also associated with risk for hypogonadism. Androgen deficiency can occur in both men and women following opioid use and lead to depression-like symptoms such as fatigue, sleeping too much, and low libido.[55,56] Additional research is needed to determine if androgen deficiency-related mood disturbance resolves after opioid cessation and whether testosterone replacement therapy relieves depression symptoms. Whether opioid-induced androgen deficiency is a key mechanism or part of a constellation of factors contributing to new-onset depression following LTOT has yet to be determined.

Occupation of opioid receptors by prescription opioids over a long period may cause downregulation in the number of opioid receptors, leading to a reduced capacity for persons to experience natural reward and maintain hedonic capacity. As discussed in Chapter 2, chronic opioid use can lead to changes in neurophysiology that remain long after opioid use has stopped. The neuroanatomical changes following opioid use support the evidence that depression is not a side effect of LTOT, but, instead, LTOT is associated with increased risk for new-onset depression even after opioid cessation. One likely mechanism for the association between prescription opioid use and depression are the opioid-related neurophysiological changes in parts of the brain responsible for experiencing reward and pleasure.

4.16 Psychosocial Mechanisms

Although opioid use disorder does not explain the association between frequent opioid use in LTOT and new-onset depression, patients who develop problem opioid use are also more likely to experience a host of adverse life events that may impact depression risk. Symptoms of opioid use disorder such as borrowing medication from friends or family and/or losing control over opioids are correlated with divorce, separation, job loss, unemployment, decreased physical activity, and social isolation.[57,58] These psychosocial factors are common in depression, and they may be factors underlying the link between LTOT and new-onset depression.

LTOT remains associated with new-onset depression after accounting for numerous pain conditions and pain severity.[4] However, pain interference may explain more variance in depression risk than does pain severity. *Pain interference* refers to limitations in patients' ability to participate in self-care, work, and social activities. Increasing social isolation may follow, which in turn can worsen depression symptoms.[59,60] It is possible that pain interference and not perceived pain severity mediates the relationship between LTOT and depression.

4.17 Public Health and Clinical Relevance

Based on 2018 data, about 18% of adults in the United States received an opioid prescription in the past year.[61] Of these, 4–5%, will become greater than 90-day users. Based on a conservative estimate of the magnitude of association between LTOT and new-onset depression, just 12 non-cancer pain patients would need to have more than 90-day opioid use to generate one depression case. This equates to 156,000 new depression cases that onset in middle-age and might not have occurred if LTOT was avoided. Given the enormous burden of depression, avoiding LTOT could improve population mental health. Since 2012, the rate of opioid prescribing in the United States has declined, yet patients with versus without risk factors (e.g., depression, anxiety, substance use disorders) for adverse opioid outcomes continue to be more likely to be prescribed an opioid.[62] More careful selection of patients for opioid therapy is needed.

Clinicians and patients should be educated about the association between LTOT and new-onset depression. While it is recommended that patients be screened for depression and other psychiatric disorders before starting an opioid, the research discussed here indicates that repeated depression screening should be done with patients receiving LTOT. Patients who report that their depression is due to their pain should be counseled that their depression may be due to LTOT. Patients may report short-term improvement in mood after starting an opioid, but clinicians and patients should be aware of the risk for worsening mood following chronic opioid use. Last, because more frequent opioid use is associated with new-onset depression,[13] patients should be advised to try to limit the number of days they use an opioid to avoid increasing the risk for depression.

4.18 Conclusion

There is considerable evidence that LTOT is followed by new depressive episodes. Future studies need to determine if the risk is specific to depression or if the risk increases for multiple mood disorders such as dysthymia. The Prescription Opioids and Depression Pathways Cohort study is currently under way. Participants are all starting a new period of 30- to 90-day prescription opioid use at baseline.[63,64] Lifetime histories of depression and dysthymia are being collected as are measures of anhedonia and vital exhaustion. Once follow-up is complete, it will be possible to determine if patients free of a lifetime history of depression are at elevated risk of developing any depression symptoms and DSM-5 criteria depression following LTOT. In addition to establishing the strongest evidence for whether LTOT leads to depression, this study will identify any moderators and mediators of the opioid–depression relationship. If confirmed, pragmatic trials that proactively screen for depression and treat depression to remission as part of LTOT should be conducted to determine if this risk can be averted among patients in need of opioid therapy.

References

1. Goldner EM, Lusted A, Roerecke M, Rehm J, Fischer B. Prevalence of Axis-1 psychiatric (with focus on depression and anxiety) disorder and symptomatology among non-medical prescription opioid users in substance use treatment: Systematic review and meta-analyses. *Addict Behav.* 2014;39(3):520–531.
2. van Rijswijk SM, van Beek M, Schoof GM, Schene AH, Steegers M, Schellekens AF. Iatrogenic opioid use disorder, chronic pain and psychiatric comorbidity: A systematic review. *Gen Hosp Psychiatry.* 2019;59:37–50.
3. Barry DT, Cutter CJ, Beitel M, Kerns RD, Liong C, Schottenfeld RS. Psychiatric disorders among patients seeking treatment for co-occurring chronic pain and opioid use disorder. *J Clin Psychiatry.* 2016;77(10):1413–1419.
4. Scherrer JF, Salas J, Copeland LA, et al. Prescription opioid duration, dose, and increased risk of depression in 3 large patient populations. *Annals of Family Medicine.* 2016;14:54–62.
5. Scherrer JF, Svrakic DM, Freedland KE, et al. Prescription opioid analgesics increase the risk of depression. *J Gen Intern Med.* 2014;29(3):491–499.
6. International Association for the Study of Pain. Acute pain. https://www.iasp-pain.org/resources/topics/acute-pain/ Accessed Dec. 1, 2022.
7. Treede RD, Rief W, Barke A, et al. A classification of chronic pain for ICD-11. *Pain.* 2015;156(6):1003–1007.
8. Stevans JM, Delitto A, Khoja SS, et al. Risk factors associated with transition from acute to chronic low back pain in US patients seeking primary care. *JAMA Network Open.* 2021;4(2):e2037371.
9. Von Korff M, Shortreed SM, LeResche L, et al. A longitudinal study of depression among middle-aged and senior patients initiating chronic opioid therapy. *J Affect Disord.* 2017;211:136–143.
10. Smith K, Mattick RP, Bruno R, et al. Factors associated with the development of depression in chronic non-cancer pain patients following the onset of opioid treatment for pain. *J Affect Disord.* 2015;184:72–80.
11. Seal KH, Shi Y, Cohen G, et al. Association of mental health disorders with prescription opioids and high-risk opioid use in US Veterans of Iraq and Afghanistan. *JAMA.* 2012;307:940–947.
12. Edlund MJ, Martin BC, Fan MY, Devries A, Braden JB, Sullivan MD. Risks for opioid abuse and dependence among recipients of chronic opioid therapy: Results from the TROUP study. *Drug Alcohol Depend.* 2010;112(1–2):90–98.

RISK 59

13. Scherrer JF, Salas J, Miller-Matero LR, et al. Long-term Prescription Opioid Users Risk for New Onset Depression Increases with Frequency of Use. *Pain.* 2022 Aug 1;163(8):1581–1589.

14. Salas J, Scherrer JF, Schneider FD, et al. New-onset depression following stable, slow, and rapid rate of prescription opioid dose escalation. *Pain.* 2017;158(2):306–312.

15. Boudreau D, Von Korff M, Rutter CM, et al. Trends in long-term opioid therapy for chronic non-cancer pain. *Pharmacoepidemiol Drug Safety.* 2009;18(12):1166–1175.

16. Von Korff M, Saunders K, Thomas Ray G, et al. De facto long-term opioid therapy for noncancer pain. *Clin J Pain.* 2008;24(6):521–527.

17. Ostling PS, Davidson KS, Anyama BO, Helander EM, Wyche MQ, Kaye AD. America's opioid epidemic: A comprehensive review and look into the rising crisis. *Curr Pain Headache Rep.* 2018;22(5):1–7.

18. Kroenke K, Wu J, Bair MJ, Krebs EE, Damush TM, Tu W. Reciprocal relationship between pain and depression: A 12-month longitudinal analysis in primary care. *J Pain.* 2011;12:964–973.

19. Bair MJ, Robinson RL, Katon W, Kroenke K. Depression and pain comorbidity: A literature review. *Arch Intern Med.* 2003;163(20):2433–2445.

20. Sullivan MD, Ballantyne JC. What are we treating with long-term opioid therapy? *Arch Intern Med.* 2012;172(5):433–434.

21. Sullivan MD. Why does depression promote long-term opioid use? *Pain.* 2016;157(11):2395–2396.

22. Austin PC, Stuart EA. Moving towards best practice when using inverse probability of treatment weighting (IPTW) using the propensity score to estimate causal treatment effects in observational studies. *Stat Med.* 2015;34:3661–3679.

23. Austin PC. Balance diagnostics for comparing the distribution of baseline covariates between treatment groups in propensity-score matched samples. *Stat Med.* 2009;28(25):3083–3107.

24. Scherrer JF, Salas J, Sullivan MD, et al. The influence of prescription opioid use duration and dose on development of treatment resistant depression. *Prev Med.* 2016;91:110–116.

25. Scherrer JF, Salas J, Copeland LA, et al. Increased risk of depression recurrence after initiation of prescription opioids in noncancer pain patients. *J Pain.* 2016;17(4):473–482.

26. Merrill JO, Von Korff M, Banta-Green CJ, et al. Prescribed opioid difficulties, depression and opioid dose among chronic opioid therapy patients. *Gen Hosp Psychiatry.* 2012;34(6):581–587.

27. Hong N, Jung MH, Kim JW, et al. Opioid analgesics and depressive symptoms in burn patients: What is the real relationship? *Clin Psychopharmacol Neurosci.* 2016;14(3):295–298.

28. Kroenke K, Strine TW, Spitzer RL, Williams JB, Berry JT, Mokdad AH. The PHQ-8 as a measure of current depression in the general population. *J Affect Disord.* 2009;114(1–3):163–173.

29. Trevino CM, Brasel K. Does opiate use in traumatically injured individuals worsen pain and psychological outcomes? *J Pain.* 2013;14(4):424–430.

30. Solberg LI, Engebretson KI, Sperl-Hillen JM, Hroscikoski MC, O'Connor PG. Are claims data accurate enough to identify patients for performance measures or quality improvement? The case of diabetes, heart disease and depression. *Am J Med Qual.* 2006;21:238–245.

31. Frayne SM, Miller DR, Sharkansky EJ, et al. Using administrative data to identify mental illness: What approach is best? *Am J Med Qual.* 2010;25(1):42–50.

32. Gravely AA, Cutting A, Nugent S, Grill J, Carlson K, Spoont M. Validity of PTSD diagnoses in VA administrative data: Comparison of VA administrative PTSD diagnoses to self-reported PTSD Checklist scores. *J Rehabil Res Dev.* 2011;48(1):21–30.

33. Holowka DW, Marx BP, Gates MA, et al. PTSD diagnostic validity in Veterans Affairs electronic records of Iraq and Afghanistan veterans. *J Consult Clin Psychol.* 2014;82(4):569–579.

34. Quintana MI, Mari Jde J, Ribeiro WS, Jorge MR, Andreoli SB. Accuracy of the Composite International Diagnostic Interview (CIDI 2.1) for diagnosis of post-traumatic stress disorder according to DSM-IV criteria. *Cad Saude Publica.* 2012;28(7):1312–1318.
35. Kimerling R, Serpi T, Weathers F, et al. Diagnostic accuracy of the Composite International Diagnostic Interview (CIDI 3.0) PTSD module among female Vietnam-era veterans. *J Trauma Stress.* 2014;27(2):160–167.
36. Haneuse S, VanderWeele TJ, Arterburn D. Using the e-value to assess the potential effect of unmeasured confounding in observational studies. *JAMA.* 2019;321(6):602–603.
37. Scherrer JF, Salas J, Copeland LA, et al. Prescription opioid duration, dose, and increased risk of depression in 3 large patient populations. *Ann Fam Med.* 2016;14(1):54–62.
38. Scherrer JF, Salas J, Copeland LA, et al. Increased risk of depression recurrence after initiation of prescription opioids in non-cancer pain patients. *J Pain.* 2016;17:473–482.
39. Salas J, Scherrer JF, Ahmedani BK, et al. Gender and the association between long-term prescription opioid use and new-onset depression. *J Pain.* 2018;19(1):88–98.
40. Wilson L, Bekeris J, Fiasconaro M, et al. Risk factors for new-onset depression or anxiety following total joint arthroplasty: The role of chronic opioid use. *Reg Anesth Pain Med.* 2019 Sep 16:rapm-2019-100785.
41. Scherrer JF, Salas J, Lustman PJ, Burge S, Schneider FD. Change in opioid dose and change in depression in a longitudinal primary care patient cohort. *Pain.* 2015;156:348–355.
42. Scherrer JF, Salas J, Lustman PJ, Burge S, Schneider FD, Residency Research Network of Texas I. Change in opioid dose and change in depression in a longitudinal primary care patient cohort. *Pain.* 2015;156(2):348–355.
43. Ballantyne JC, Sullivan MD, Koob GF. Refractory dependence on opioid analgesics. *Pain.* 2019;160(12):2655–2660.
44. Shurman J, Koob GF, Gutstein HB. Opioids, pain, the brain, and hyperkatifeia: A framework for the rational use of opioids for pain. *Pain Med.* 2010;11(7):1092–1098.
45. Garfield JBB, Cotton SM, Allen NB, et al. Evidence that anhedonia is a symptom of opioid dependence associated with recent use. *Drug Alcohol Depend.* 2017;177:29–38.
46. Garland EL, Trostheim M, Eikemo M, Ernst G, Leknes S. Anhedonia in chronic pain and prescription opioid misuse. *Psychol Med.* 2020;50(12):1977–1988.
47. Hill AB. The environment and disease: Association or causation? *Proc R Soc Med.* 1965;58:295–300.
48. Katikireddi SV, Green MJ, Taylor AE, Davey Smith G, Munafo MR. Assessing causal relationships using genetic proxies for exposures: An introduction to Mendelian randomization. *Addiction.* 2018;113(4):764–774.
49. Rosoff DB, Smith GD, Lohoff FW. Prescription opioid use and risk for major depressive disorder and anxiety and stress-related disorders: A multivariable mendelian randomization analysis. *JAMA Psychiatry.* 2021;78(2):151–160.
50. Filiatrault ML, Chauny JM, Daoust R, Roy MP, Denis R, Lavigne G. Medium increased risk for central sleep apnea but not obstructive sleep apnea in long-term opioid users: A systematic review and meta-analysis. *J Clin Sleep Med.* 2016;12(4):617–625.
51. Morasco BJ, O'Hearn D, Turk DC, Dobscha SK. Associations between prescription opioid use and sleep impairment among veterans with chronic pain. *Pain Med.* 2014;15(11):1902–1910.
52. Zhang MM, Ma Y, Du LT, et al. Sleep disorders and non-sleep circadian disorders predict depression: A systematic review and meta-analysis of longitudinal studies. *Neurosci Biobehav Rev.* 2022;134:104532.
53. Salas J, Miller MB, Scherrer JF, et al. The association of opioid use duration and new depression episode among patients with and without insomnia. *J Opioid Manag.* 2020;16(5):317–328.
54. Lee M, Silverman SM, Hansen H, Patel VB, Manchikanti L. A comprehensive review of opioid-induced hyperalgesia. *Pain Physician.* 2011;14(2):145–161.

55. Smith HS, Elliott JA. Opioid-induced androgen deficiency (OPIAD). *Pain Physician.* 2012;15:ES145–ES156.
56. Elliott JA, Horton E, Fibuch EE. The endocrine effects of long-term oral opioid therapy: A case report and review of the literature. *J Opioid Manage.* 2011;7(2):145–154.
57. Blanco C, Wiley TRA, Lloyd JJ, Lopez MF, Volkow ND. America's opioid crisis: The need for an integrated public health approach. *Transl Psychiatry.* 2020;10(1):167.
58. Salmond S, Allread V. A population health approach to America's opioid epidemic. *Orthop Nurs.* 2019;38(2):95–108.
59. Bannon S, Greenberg J, Mace RA, Locascio JJ, Vranceanu AM. The role of social isolation in physical and emotional outcomes among patients with chronic pain. *Gen Hosp Psychiatry.* 2021;69:50–54.
60. Penacoba Puente C, Velasco Furlong L, Ecija Gallardo C, Cigaran Mendez M, Bedmar Cruz D, Fernandez-de-Las-Penas C. Self-efficacy and affect as mediators between pain dimensions and emotional symptoms and functional limitation in women with fibromyalgia. *Pain Manag Nurs.* 2015;16(1):60–68.
61. NORC. One-third of Americans have received an opioid prescription in the past two years. https://www.norc.org/NewsEventsPublications/PressReleases/Pages/one-third-of-americans-have-received-an-opioid-prescription-in-the-past-two-years.aspx Accessed Feb. 27, 2023.
62. Scherrer JF, Tucker J, Salas J, Zhang Z, Grucza R. Comparison of opioids prescribed for patients at risk for opioid misuse before and after publication of the Centers for Disease Control and Prevention's Opioid Prescribing Guidelines. *JAMA Network Open.* 2020;3(12):e2027481.
63. Salas J, Scherrer JF, Tuerk P, et al. Large posttraumatic stress disorder improvement and antidepressant medication adherence. *J Affect Disord.* 2020;260:119–123.
64. Secrest S, Miller-Matero LR, Chrusciel T, et al. Baseline characteristics from a new longitudinal cohort of patients with noncancer pain and chronic opioid use in the United States. *J Pain.* 2023. Oct 30:S1526–5900(23)00595-3.

5

Depression and Pain

Bidirectional Relationship and Changes with Psychological Treatment

Lisa R. Miller-Matero

5.1 Introduction

Individuals with a chronic pain condition are at risk of experiencing psychiatric distress. For example, those with chronic pain experience mood and anxiety disorders at approximately twice the rate as the general population.[1] As many as 50% of individuals with chronic pain meet criteria for a depressive disorder, and 35% meet criteria for an anxiety disorder.[2] Moreover, severity of pain and mental health symptoms are linked, such that those with greater pain severity report higher levels of depression and anxiety.[3-6]

In addition to pain severity, other pain-related factors are associated with mental health, including pain interference and pain catastrophizing. *Pain interference* is the degree to which pain affects individual's activities of daily living, such as work, social activities, and household chores.[7] Pain severity is not always associated with the degree to which pain interferes with functioning, and depression may explain this relationship.[8] The directionality of depression and pain interference is unclear, however. Some work has suggested that greater pain interference increases risk for a depression diagnosis.[9] Other studies suggest the relationship may be in the opposite direction and find that greater depression was associated with greater pain interference[10]; although depression predicted pain interference, pain interference did not predict depression.[11] Yet there is also the possibility of a bidirectional effect. One study not only found that individuals with probable depression at a baseline assessment predicted the development of pain interference 3 years later (odds ratio [OR] = 2.42; 95% confidence interval [CI]: 1.24, 4.69), they also found that pain interference at the baseline assessment also increased risk for having depression 3 years later (OR = 2.47;

Lisa R. Miller-Matero, *Depression and Pain* In: *Pain, the Opioid Epidemic, & Depression*. Edited by: Jeffrey F. Scherrer & Jane C. Ballantyne, Oxford University Press. © Oxford University Press 2024. DOI: 10.1093/9780197675250.003.0005

CI: 1.96, 3.11).[12] Although the findings regarding the directionality of pain interference and depression are mixed, it is clear that there is a strong association between these factors.

Pain catastrophizing occurs when an individual magnifies the negative experience of pain.[13] In pain catastrophizing, the individual will feel helpless and ruminate about the pain. Pain catastrophizing is often measured with the Pain Catastrophizing Scale, and some examples of items from this scale, which suggest catastrophizing thoughts, include "I worry all the time about whether the pain will end," "I can't seem to keep it out of my mind," and "There is nothing I can do to reduce the intensity of the pain."[13] Pain catastrophizing is associated with adjustment to having a chronic pain condition. A meta-analysis found that individuals with high levels of pain catastrophizing were at increased risk for greater pain severity and pain interference.[14] In addition, higher levels of pain catastrophizing are also associated with depression.[15]

Taken together, chronic pain is a frequent and costly health complaint, and depression commonly occurs among individuals with pain. In addition, there is a bidirectional relationship between depression and the experience of chronic pain. Given this strong relationship between pain and depression, and the impact that these have on the individual and society, it is essential that these factors be treated simultaneously.

5.2 Psychological Treatments for Co-Occurring Chronic Pain and Depression

The recognition that pain and depression co-occur has led to the development and evaluation of psychological interventions that simultaneously target both depression and pain. Because negative mood is likely to affect treatment motivation and adherence with treatment recommendations among individuals with chronic pain, it is important to address depression within pain treatment.[16] A variety of theoretical orientations have been used to develop strategies to treat comorbid depression and pain. The interventions that have been most commonly used and tested include cognitive behavioral therapy (CBT), mindfulness, and acceptance and commitment therapy (ACT). Common components within each of these interventions are highlighted in Table 5.1.

64 LISA R. MILLER-MATERO

Table 5.1 Examples of common components utilized in psychological treatments to manage co-occurring chronic pain and depression

Cognitive Behavioral Therapy (CBT)
Psychoeducation
Relaxation
Reframing thoughts
Behavioral activation
Pacing
Mindfulness
Mindfulness meditation
Body scan
Progressive muscle relaxation
Guided imagery
Leaves on a stream
Acceptance and Commitment Therapy (ACT)
Avoidance vs. acceptance
Cognitive defusion
Contact with the present moment
Committed action
Values-based action

5.2.1 Cognitive Behavioral Therapy

CBT is arguably the most frequently tested modality for chronic pain management. CBT focuses on the relationships among thoughts, emotions, and behaviors and how these interact.[17] CBT is an effective treatment for improving depression[18] and can be similarly applied in the treatment of pain. As mentioned, there is an association between thoughts (i.e., catastrophizing) and emotions (i.e., depression) with the pain experience (i.e., pain severity and interference with daily activities). Within CBT, a variety of strategies can be used to assist individuals in managing pain. Psychoeducation is commonly used in CBT for pain, including an explanation of how thoughts, emotions, and behaviors interact and influence each other to affect the pain experience. The biopsychosocial concept of pain and the gate control theory of pain can be used by clinicians to explain how the pain experience is determined by factors beyond simple signal transmission.[16,19] Providing

DEPRESSION AND PAIN   65

this information to patients may improve knowledge about why psychological interventions can be helpful. CBT may be effective because it helps a patient alter their pain beliefs. Individuals with chronic pain often have misconstrued beliefs about the cause and course of their pain,[20] and these pain beliefs are related to their adjustment to chronic pain.[21,22] Beliefs about pain, such as that pain is a signal of damage, that it can lead to disability, that it is uncontrollable, and that activity should be avoided, have been shown to be maladaptive in dealing with pain.[21,22] In CBT for pain, the therapist can help the patient identify and change any negative or inaccurate thoughts and emotions surrounding the experience of pain.[17,23] Altering thoughts about the pain experience can lead to better pain outcomes.[24] In addition, *pain reprocessing therapy* (PRT) is a more recent psychological treatment that focuses on addressing the fear and misbeliefs about pain. This treatment has been successful in shifting the beliefs about pain resulting from tissue damage to attributing pain to mind/brain factors[25] and has shown substantial improvement in pain.[26]

In addition to identifying and reframing thoughts, several other CBT strategies commonly are used as a part of pain management. Relaxation is a strategy used for decades in the management of chronic pain.[27] Practicing relaxation is helpful for pain.[28,29] Teaching patients how to engage in relaxation has been helpful in increasing the use of relaxation skills[28] as well as in improving pain coping skills,[28] pain severity,[29] distress,[29,30] sleep,[29] and quality of life.[29]

Individuals with chronic pain may avoid engaging in activities for fear of worsening pain.[31] This avoidance of activity is related to poorer functioning for individuals with chronic pain, including greater anxiety and disability and lower levels of activity.[32–34] Those who engage in little avoidance and maintain high levels of activity have demonstrated the best outcomes,[34] suggesting that encouraging physical activity among individuals with pain may be useful in increasing their functioning. Thus, behavioral activation is another common strategy used within CBT, which encourages individuals to engage in regular, pleasurable activities. Behavioral activation is helpful for depression,[35] and it can improve pain-related outcomes among individuals with chronic pain.[36] Within pain treatment, behavioral activation is often paired with pacing. *Pacing* encourages individuals to engage in regular activities without over-engagement. Individuals engaging in behavioral activation while pacing their activities experienced improvements in

66 LISA R. MILLER-MATERO

anxiety and depression and decreased medication usage and interference with daily activities.[36]

5.2.2 Mindfulness

Mindfulness is another modality garnering support for co-occurring chronic pain management and depression. Mindfulness is being in the present moment and being aware of one's own thoughts and emotions without judgment; it has been used with individuals with medical illness, including pain.[37,38] Within mindfulness, many different strategies can be used to help an individual practice being in a mindful state. *Guided imagery* is a common strategy used in mindfulness practice. Guided imagery is often composed of words and/or music and is meant to elicit a positive scene or situation in which various senses are evoked.[39] Common scenes include being at a beach or in a forest. Guided imagery may lower ratings of pain severity, reduce the degree to which pain interferes in daily functioning, and improves symptoms of depression.[39-41] In conducting a *body scan*, an individual will focus on various parts of their body and notice, without judgment, how that body part feels. A body scan can offer immediate improvements in ratings of pain severity, interference in daily activities, and mood.[42] *Progressive muscle relaxation* takes a body scan one step further. During progressive muscle relaxation, an individual concentrates on various parts of the body, but also contracts and releases each muscle group. Practicing progressive muscle relaxation may reduce pain severity and interference in daily activities.[43] A final example of a mindfulness strategy is recognizing thoughts, but letting them pass. Using analogies is common in mindfulness practice: "leaves on a stream" is an example of a metaphor used in this practice (i.e., identifying that the thoughts are occurring but letting them pass like leaves carried on a stream).[44] Mindfulness strategies can be delivered on their own or through a full course of treatment (i.e., mindfulness-based stress reduction). *Mindfulness-based stress reduction* is commonly delivered across eight (1.5- to 2-hour) sessions and can reduce pain severity and interference in daily activities and improve quality of life among individuals with low back pain.[45] More broadly, in a systematic review, mindfulness meditation has been found to lead to statistically significant improvements for pain severity, pain interference, pain catastrophizing, quality of life, anxiety, and depression.[24,46-48]

5.2.3 Acceptance and Commitment Therapy

A third modality commonly used for management of chronic pain and depression is acceptance and commitment therapy (ACT). ACT is composed of mindfulness strategies, but extends mindfulness by teaching the patient how to be psychologically flexible through pain acceptance, cognitive defusion, committed action, and values-based action.[49,50] Becoming psychologically flexible allows individuals to accept their thoughts and behaviors and engage in value-based activities despite having chronic pain.[51-53] The concept of avoidance is often discussed, including the potential negative impact that avoidance can have on pain outcomes. In contrast, the benefits of accepting the pain are taught, as pain acceptance is associated with less depression and better pain outcomes (i.e., lower pain severity and pain interference).[54] Values-based action is often included within ACT. Individuals with chronic pain may not be engaging in activities they previously valued due to their pain; clinicians can assist in identifying the individual's values and ways in which the individual can engage in activities that align with their values. Engaging in values-based action promotes better outcomes such as pain acceptance, psychological flexibility, pain interference, and mood.[50]

Individuals who are mindful and are accepting of their pain report lower pain severity, distress, and disability.[37,55-59] These techniques may have an indirect effect on pain by altering anxiety sensitivity, which is related to greater pain, disability, and distress.[60] ACT is associated with improvements in pain severity, anxiety, depression, pain interference, pain catastrophizing, and satisfaction with life.[30] In a meta-analysis, mindfulness and ACT interventions demonstrated small effect sizes for depression and pain severity and moderate effect sizes for anxiety and pain interference.[61] In addition, ACT exhibited a stronger effect for depression and anxiety than mindfulness-based interventions; however, mindfulness and ACT may have outcomes comparable to CBT.[61]

5.3 Psychological Interventions to Reduce Prescription Opioid Use Among Individuals with Chronic Pain

Prescription opioids have been commonly used in the management of chronic pain; however, long-term use of opioids is now strongly discouraged because of the increased risk of an opioid use disorder, overdose, and death.[62] Individuals with depression are at higher risk for transitioning to long-term opioid use compared to those without depression.[63] This could be because those with depression do not receive the same analgesic benefit from opioids compared to those without depression, or those with depression may be using opioids for reasons other than pain management (i.e., to assist with sleep or stress management).[64] On the other hand, long-term opioid use is also linked with increased risk for depression, which supports the potential for a bidirectional relationship between opioid use and depression.[65]

Unfortunately, tapering opioid prescriptions is challenging, and more than half of individuals prescribed opioids for 3 months are still using opioids up to 5 years later.[66] Abrupt cessation of opioids, especially when involuntary, can be harmful, with increased risk of withdrawal, overdose, emergency department visits, or inpatient admissions.[67-69] It may be especially difficult to reduce opioid use among individuals with depression because those with depression may have impaired motivation and are more likely to experience higher pain severity and interference in daily activities.[3-6,8,70] Thus, psychological interventions may not only be effective for managing pain, but could also offer support in reducing opioid use. Preliminary evidence from small trials suggest that similar treatment modalities used for pain management could be applied to opioid cessation programs (i.e., CBT, mindfulness, and ACT). Among individuals with chronic pain and long-term use, CBT, mindfulness, and acceptance-based strategies are associated with reduced opioid use.[71-74] Mindfulness and CBT approaches have also been piloted among those who have chronic pain and opioid misuse. These interventions appear feasible and have reduced desire for opioids, opioid use, and risk of developing an opioid use disorder.[75,76] However, given that these interventions are in their infancy, larger trials are needed to better understand how psychological interventions influence opioid use.

5.4 Challenges in Managing Comorbid Pain, Depression, and Opioid Use and Potential Solutions

Despite promising studies of psychological interventions for chronic pain management, there are several challenges. First, effect sizes tend to be modest for most outcomes. Most psychological interventions for chronic pain show improvement among pain-related and psychological-related variables, yet meta-analyses have generally found small to medium effect sizes across various outcomes.[61,77,78] In addition, various psychological interventions for chronic pain management appear to perform similarly in improving chronic pain and related distress.[61] Thus, it is unclear which components of the interventions are useful and which components are beneficial for pain-related factors, psychological factors, or both. More work to identify the helpful components could assist in developing person-centered treatments. This could result in a tailored application of components for each individual, which could lead to greater treatment effects. Second, most research on psychological interventions for chronic pain has been with White, middle- to upper-class individuals. Generalizability of these interventions to other racial and ethnic groups is unknown. Cultural beliefs about pain and distress could impact outcomes, and, as such, adaptations to existing interventions may be needed. Third, there are only pilot trials examining these interventions for opioid use as an outcome.[71-73,75,76] Although these pilot trials show promise for improving pain outcomes and opioid use, much more research is needed with larger sample sizes that can also examine mechanisms. It is also likely that, to have maximum impact on pain and opioid use, psychological interventions need to be combined or integrated with other evidence-based treatments.

In addition to challenges with the interventions themselves, it has also been difficult to engage patients in psychological interventions for pain management. Primary care providers report that they lack nonpharmacological treatment options to refer patients to.[79] Providers also report that if patients are already receiving opioids, they seem less interested in engaging in nonpharmacological approaches. Even if providers do refer, it is often to a general mental health clinic, where most clinicians do not have training or expertise in managing co-occurring chronic pain and distress. Patient-related factors that interfere with engagement in psychological interventions for chronic pain include physical limitations to ambulate to appointments, transportation, low motivation, cost, and time constraints.[80,81] Indeed, most existing treatments are lengthy, most often ranging from 8–12 sessions that are 1–2 hours each.[45,61,75,76,82] As such, premature dropout from treatment is also common.[83,84]

Methods being piloted to increase treatment initiation and adherence to psychological interventions for chronic pain include offering treatment through primary care, developing brief interventions, and providing options to attend appointments via telemedicine. Because pain is one of the most common reasons individuals see a primary care provider[85] and accounts for approximately 40% of all primary care visits,[86] engaging patients in an intervention in a primary care setting may be useful. Integrating behavioral health providers in primary care has been a growing model of care, including behavioral health consultant and collaborative care models. These models have behavioral health providers located in primary care clinics and/or as direct referrals from primary care. Integrating clinicians in primary care increases patient access and utilization of general mental health services, including treatment for depression.[87–93] This increase in access and utilization occurs regardless of gender,[87] race/ethnicity,[87,94] age,[87] and insurance type.[88] Offering integrated care also results in fewer missed appointments,[87,88] which could lead to a lower dropout rate among individuals receiving psychological treatments for chronic pain. Importantly, patients and providers are highly satisfied with integrated primary care services.[89,95–100] Individuals report having better access to care,[95] perceive their care as better coordinated,[95,98,99] and feel as though they are being treated from a more holistic perspective.[96,97]

Although there are existing integrated models in primary care where psychological interventions for chronic pain could be delivered, a limitation is that current interventions for pain are lengthier than the integrated models currently allow. As mentioned, most interventions that have been tested require 8–12 sessions (1–2 hours each),[45,61,75,76,82] whereas many integrated primary care models use time-limited, brief treatments (i.e., 4–6 sessions, 30 minutes each). A briefer psychological intervention has been developed to be delivered through existing integrated models and has been evaluated through a pilot trial. In the pilot, the intervention showed promise for reducing pain severity, pain interference, pain catastrophizing, and depression at post-intervention.[101] A 6-month follow-up also suggested similar long-term effects to lengthier interventions.[102] Finally, this intervention also showed promise for influencing opioid use.[74] However, it is important to note that this intervention has only been tested through a pilot randomized controlled trial, and it should be tested through a fully powered clinical trial.

A final method that can be used to increase engagement in a psychological intervention for chronic pain is utilization of telemedicine. Conducting visits virtually can eliminate some of the common barriers that interfere with engagement because it eliminates the need for transportation, can lower costs for patients, and may require a lower time commitment compared to in-person treatments. Individuals with chronic pain are satisfied with a telemedicine delivery of services,[103] and such services are desirable even among older adults (e.g., 60 and older).[104] Thus, it appears that virtual visits are feasible and acceptable for the delivery of psychological interventions for pain management. However, some individuals may prefer in-person appointments within an integrated care model,[105] and so it is important to consider patient preferences.

5.5 Conclusion

There are several potential areas for future work regarding the treatment of co-occurring chronic pain and depression. As mentioned, more work is needed to better engage individuals in interventions and also further test interventions for efficacy in improving pain, distress, and opioid use. Combining psychological strategies with other evidence-based treatments may improve outcomes. In addition, research could also begin to develop culturally adapted versions of these interventions as needed. Existing interventions have mostly been tested on middle- to upper-class White women, and greater diversity is needed to determine whether these interventions are equitable for individuals from other sociodemographic backgrounds. Individuals from certain racial and ethnic groups report significantly higher pain severity than do White patients[106]; however, some racial and ethnic groups (Black, Hispanic, Asian) are less likely to be treated with opioids,[106-108] less likely to be referred to specialty pain management services,[108,109] and more likely to have inadequate pain management.[110] Black patients are also more likely to wait longer to request pain management, and, when they do seek treatment, Black patients are more likely to have their pain undertreated.[110,111] Compounding this, historically marginalized groups are less likely to engage in mental health services, which could be because of poor access to providers, attitudes toward mental health services, or stigma.[112-114] Taken together, some individuals are at higher risk for poorer outcomes, yet it is not clear whether existing interventions are efficacious for all patients or whether adaptations to treatments are needed.

Research can also continue to identify novel methods to engage individuals in treatment. Delivery through telemedicine may increase uptake of interventions. In addition to virtual visits, self-guided applications or web-based applications have shown promise for improving outcomes and may provide avenues to increase engagement and adherence to treatment.[115] Although primary care appears to be a setting that can successfully engage patients, other medical settings can be used to deliver interventions as well, such as physical therapy, orthopedics, and pain clinics. In addition, interventions could be delivered as a preventive measure. Factors associated with risk of transition from acute pain to chronic pain include low mood, depression, anxiety, and/or higher levels of pain catastrophizing.[116-120] Similar factors are also associated with greater risk of developing prolonged opioid use. Specifically, physical (i.e., pain intensity, pain interference) and affective factors (i.e., depression) are related to a higher likelihood of patients continuing on opioids.[121,122] Delivering interventions to high-risk individuals could prevent the transition to chronic pain and long-term opioid use. Several psychological interventions have been delivered prior to a surgical procedure and were associated with lower postoperative pain severity.[123,124] However, it is not yet clear whether these interventions could reduce postoperative opioid use. In addition, a remaining gap exists for those who experience an unexpected injury or do not have the opportunity to complete a preoperative intervention, although some pilot work shows promise for psychological interventions delivered postoperatively to reduce acute pain as well.[125] Thus, there is a need for effective postoperative interventions that could reduce the likelihood of transitioning from acute to chronic pain as well as prolonged opioid use.

A final future direction to consider is the need for policy changes. Many individuals with chronic pain face barriers to utilizing care, which could include limits on number of sessions, access to virtual care, or costly co-pays. Furthermore, billing for integrated services presents its own challenges. The most common financial barriers include the separation of physical and behavioral health payment structures, problems coding for behavioral health consultant services in primary care, difficulties with reimbursement using Health and Behavior Assessment codes, issues with same-day billing from multiple providers, poor reimbursement rates, and lack of reimbursement for collaborative care.[126-131]

In conclusion, the development of psychological treatments for co-occurring chronic pain and depression began decades ago, and many strategies within these treatments produce benefits for psychological factors and pain-related outcomes. However, there is still a great deal of work to do to increase effects of the interventions, engage individuals in treatment, and ensure equitable care.

References

1. McWilliams LA, Cox BJ, Enns MW. Mood and anxiety disorders associated with chronic pain: an examination in a nationally representative sample. 2003;106(1–2):127–133.
2. Bair MJ, Wu J, Damush TM, Sutherland JM, Kroenke K. Association of depression and anxiety alone and in combination with chronic musculoskeletal pain in primary care patients. *Psychosomatic Med.* 2008;70(8):890.
3. Cano A, Johansen AB, Geisser M. Spousal congruence on disability, pain, and spouse responses to pain. *Pain.* 2004;109(3):258–265.
4. Currie SR, Wang J. Chronic back pain and major depression in the general Canadian population. *Pain.* 2004;107(1-2):54–60.
5. Leonard MT, Cano A, Johansen AB. Chronic pain in a couples context: A review and integration of theoretical models and empirical evidence. *J Pain.* 2006;7(6):377–390.
6. Miller LR, Cano A. Comorbid chronic pain and depression: Who is at risk? *J Pain.* 2009;10(6):619–627.
7. Amtmann D, Cook KF, Jensen MP, et al. Development of a PROMIS item bank to measure pain interference. *Pain.* 2010;150(1):173–182.
8. Miller-Matero LR, Saulino C, Clark S, Bugenski M, Eshelman A, Eisenstein D. When treating the pain is not enough: A multidisciplinary approach for chronic pelvic pain. *Arch Women Mental Health.* 2016;19(2):349–354.
9. Rayner L, Hotopf M, Petkova H, Matcham F, Simpson A, McCracken LM. Depression in patients with chronic pain attending a specialised pain treatment centre: prevalence and impact on health care costs. *Pain.* 2016;157(7):1472.
10. Sánchez-Rodríguez E, Aragonès E, Jensen MP, et al. The role of pain-related cognitions in the relationship between pain severity, depression, and pain interference in a sample of primary care patients with both chronic pain and depression. *Pain Med.* 2020;21(10):2200–2211.
11. Lerman SF, Rudich Z, Brill S, Shalev H, Shahar G. Longitudinal associations between depression, anxiety, pain, and pain-related disability in chronic pain patients. *Psychosomatic Med.* 2015;77(3).
12. Arola H-M, Nicholls E, Mallen C, Thomas E. Self-reported pain interference and symptoms of anxiety and depression in community-dwelling older adults: Can a temporal relationship be determined? *Eur J Pain.* 2010;14(9):966–971.
13. Sullivan M, Bishop SR, Pivik J. The pain catastrophizing scale: Development and validation. *Psychol Assess.* 1995;7(4):524.
14. Martinez-Calderon J, Jensen MP, Morales-Asencio JM, Luque-Suarez A. Pain catastrophizing and function in individuals with chronic musculoskeletal pain. *Clin J Pain.* 2019;35(3):279–293.
15. Richardson EJ, Ness TJ, Doleys DM, Baños JH, Cianfrini L, Richards JS. Depressive symptoms and pain evaluations among persons with chronic pain: Catastrophizing, but not pain acceptance, shows significant effects. *Pain.* 2009;147(1-3):147–152.
16. Gatchel RJ, Peng YB, Peters ML, Fuchs PN, Turk DC. The biopsychosocial approach to chronic pain: scientific advances and future directions. *Psychol Bull.* 2007;133(4):581.
17. Ehde DM, Dillworth TM, Turner JA. Cognitive-behavioral therapy for individuals with chronic pain: Efficacy, innovations, and directions for research. *Am Psychol.* 2014;69(2):153.
18. Cuijpers P, Berking M, Andersson G, Quigley L, Kleiboer A, Dobson KS. A meta-analysis of cognitive-behavioural therapy for adult depression, alone and in comparison with other treatments. *Can J Psychiatry.* 2013;58(7):376–385.
19. Melzack R, Wall PD. Pain mechanisms: A new theory. *Surv Anesthesiol.* 1967;11(2):89–90.
20. Keefe FJ, Dunsmore J, Burnett R. Behavioral and cognitive-behavioral approaches to chronic pain: Recent advances and future directions. *J Consult Clin Psychol.* 1992;60(4):528–536.

74 LISA R. MILLER-MATERO

21. Turner JA, Jensen MP, Romano JM. Do beliefs, coping, and catastrophizing independently predict functioning in patients with chronic pain? *Pain.* 2000;85(1–2):115–125.
22. Jensen MP, Turner JA, Romano JM, Lawler BK. Relationship of pain-specific beliefs to chronic pain adjustment. *Pain.* 1994;57:301–309.
23. Thorn BE. *Cognitive Therapy for Chronic Pain: A Step-By-Step Guide.* Guilford; 2017.
24. Davis M, Zautra AJ, Wolf LD, Tennen H, Yeung EW. Mindfulness and cognitive–behavioral interventions for chronic pain: Differential effects on daily pain reactivity and stress reactivity. *J Consult Clin Psychol.* 2015;83(1):24.
25. Ashar Y, Perlis R, Liston C, Gunning F, Wager T. Effects of pain reprocessing therapy on attributed causes of chronic back pain. *J Pain.* 2022;23(5):27–28.
26. Ashar Y, Gordon A, Schubiner H, et al. Effect of pain reprocessing therapy vs placebo and usual care for patients with chronic back pain: A randomized clinical trial. *JAMA Psychiatry.* 2022;79(1):13–23.
27. Turner JA, Chapman CR. Psychological interventions for chronic pain: A critical review. I. Relaxation training and biofeedback. *Pain.* 1982;12(1):1–21.
28. Burns JW, Nielson WR, Jensen MP, Heapy A, Czlapinski R, Kerns RD. Does change occur for the reasons we think it does? A test of specific therapeutic operations during cognitive-behavioral treatment of chronic pain. *Clin J Pain.* 2015;31(7):603–611.
29. Chen YLE, Francis AJ. Relaxation and imagery for chronic, nonmalignant pain: effects on pain symptoms, quality of life, and mental health. *Pain Manage Nurs.* 2010;11(3):159–168.
30. Thorsell J, Finnes A, Dahl J, et al. A comparative study of 2 manual-based self-help interventions, acceptance and commitment therapy and applied relaxation, for persons with chronic pain. *Clin J Pain.* 2011;27(8):716–723.
31. Meulders A. From fear of movement-related pain and avoidance to chronic pain disability: A state-of-the-art review. *Curr Opin Behav Sci.* 2019;26:130–136.
32. Cane D, Nielson WR, McCarthy M, Mazmanian D. Pain-related activity patterns: measurement, interrelationships, and associations with psychosocial functioning. *Clin J Pain.* 2013;29(5):435–442.
33. Karsdorp PA, Vlaeyen JW. Active avoidance but not activity pacing is associated with disability in fibromyalgia. *Pain.* 2009;147(1):29–35.
34. McCracken LM, Samuel VM. The role of avoidance, pacing, and other activity patterns in chronic pain. *Pain.* 2007;130(1):119–125.
35. Lejuez CW, Hopko DR, Hopko SD. A brief behavioral activation treatment for depression treatment manual. *Behav Mod.* 2001;25(2):255–286.
36. Lundervold DA, Talley C, Buermann M. Effect of behavioral activation treatment on chronic fibromyalgia pain: Replication and extension. *Int J Behav Consult Ther.* 2008;4(2):146.
37. Kabat-Zinn J. An outpatient program in behavioral medicine for chronic pain patients based on the practice of mindfulness meditation: Theoretical considerations and preliminary results. *Gen Hosp Psychiatry.* 1982;4:33–47.
38. Creswell JD. Mindfulness interventions. *Ann Rev Psychol.* 2017;68:491–516.
39. Posadzki P, Ernst EJTCjop. Guided imagery for musculoskeletal pain: A systematic review. *Clin J Pain.* 2011 Sep;27(7):648–653.
40. Menzies V, Taylor AG, Bourguignon C. Effects of guided imagery on outcomes of pain, functional status, and self-efficacy in persons diagnosed with fibromyalgia. *J Altern Complement Med.* 2006 Jan–Feb;12(1):23–30.
41. Onieva-Zafra MD, García LH, del Valle MG. Effectiveness of guided imagery relaxation on levels of pain and depression in patients diagnosed with fibromyalgia. *Holistic Nurs Pract.* 2015;29(1):13–21.
42. Ussher M, Spatz A, Copland C, et al. Immediate effects of a brief mindfulness-based body scan on patients with chronic pain. *J Behav Med.* 2014;37(1):127–134.

43. Baird CL, Sands LJPMN. A pilot study of the effectiveness of guided imagery with progressive muscle relaxation to reduce chronic pain and mobility difficulties of osteoarthritis. *Pain Manag Nurs.* 2004;5(3):97–104.
44. Varra AA, Drossel C, Hayes SC. The use of metaphor to establish acceptance and mindfulness. *Clin Handb Mindfulness.* 2009:111–123.
45. Anheyer D, Haller H, Barth J, Lauche R, Dobos G, Cramer H. Mindfulness-based stress reduction for treating low back pain: A systematic review and meta-analysis. *Ann Intern Med.* 2017;166(11):799–807.
46. Cassidy EL, Atherton RJ, Robertson N, Walsh DA, Gillett R. Mindfulness, functioning and catastrophizing after multidisciplinary pain management for chronic low back pain. *Pain.* 2012;153(3):644–650.
47. Rod K. Observing the Effects Of Mindfulness-Based Meditation On Anxiety And Depression In Chronic Pain Patients. *Psychiatria Danubina.* 2015;27:209–211.
48. Hilton L, Hempel S, Ewing BA, et al. Mindfulness meditation for chronic pain: Systematic review and meta-analysis. *Ann Behav Med.* 2017;51(2):199–213.
49. McCracken LM, Vowles KE, Eccleston C. Acceptance of chronic pain: Component analysis and a revised assessment method. *Pain.* 2004;107(1):159–166.
50. Hughes LS, Clark J, Colclough JA, Dale E, McMillan D. Acceptance and commitment therapy (ACT) for chronic pain. *Clin J Pain.* 2017;33(6):552–568.
51. McCracken LM, Vowles KE. Acceptance and commitment therapy and mindfulness for chronic pain: Model, process, and progress. *Am Psychol.* 2014;69(2):178.
52. Trompetter H, Bohlmeijer E, Fox J, Schreurs K. Psychological flexibility and catastrophizing as associated change mechanisms during an online acceptance-based intervention for chronic pain. *Act With Pain.* 2014:145.
53. Scott W, Daly A, Yu L, McCracken LM. Treatment of chronic pain for adults 65 and over: Analyses of outcomes and changes in psychological flexibility following interdisciplinary acceptance and commitment therapy (ACT). *Pain Med.* 2017;18(2):252–264.
54. McCracken LM. Learning to live with the pain: Acceptance of pain predicts adjustment in persons with chronic pain. *Pain.* 1998;74(1):21–27.
55. Kabat-Zinn J, Lipworth L, Burney R. The clinical use of mindfulness meditation for the self-regulation of chronic pain. *J Behav Med.* 1985;8(2):163–190.
56. McCracken LM, Carson JW, Eccleston C, Keefe FJ. Acceptance and change in the context of chronic pain. *Pain.* 2004;109(1-2):4–7.
57. McCracken LM, Yang S. The role of values in contextual cognitive-behavioral approach to chronic pain. *Pain.* 2006;123:137–145.
58. Vowles KE, Wetherell JL, Sorrell JT. Targeting acceptance, mindfulness, and values-based action in chronic pain: Findings of two preliminary trials of an outpatient group-based intervention. *Cogn Behav Pract.* 2009;16:49–58.
59. Zautra AJ, Davis MC, Reich JW, et al. Comparison of cognitive-behavioral and mindfulness meditation interventions on adaptation to rheumatoid arthritis for patients with and without history of recurrent depression. *J Consul Clin Psychol.* 2008;76(3):408–421.
60. McCracken LM, Keogh E. Acceptance, mindfulness, and values-based action may counteract fear and avoidance of emotions in chronic pain: An analysis of anxiety sensitivity. *J Pain.* 2009;10(4):408–415.
61. Veehof MM, Trompetter H, Bohlmeijer ET, Schreurs KMG. Acceptance-and mindfulness-based interventions for the treatment of chronic pain: A meta-analytic review. *Cogn Behav Ther.* 2016;45(1):5–31.
62. Franklin GM. Opioids for chronic noncancer pain A position paper of the American Academy of Neurology. *Neurology.* 2014;83(14):1277–1284.
63. Sullivan MD. Depression effects on long-term prescription opioid use, abuse, and addiction. *Clin J Pain.* 2018;34(9):878–884.

64. Sullivan M. Why does depression promote long-term opioid use? *Pain.* 2016;157(11):2395–2396.
65. Scherrer JF, Salas J, Copeland LA, et al. Prescription opioid duration, dose, and increased risk of depression in 3 large patient populations. *Ann Fam Med.* 2016;14(1):54–62.
66. Martin BC, Fan MY, Edlund MJ, Devries A, Braden JB, Sullivan MD. Long-term chronic opioid therapy discontinuation rates from the TROUP study. *J Gen Intern Med.* 2011;26(12):1450–1457.
67. Agnoli A, Xing G, Tancredi DJ, Magnan E, Jerant A, Fenton JJ. Association of dose tapering with overdose or mental health crisis among patients prescribed long-term opioids. *JAMA.* 2021;326(5):411–419.
68. Mark TL, Parish W. Opioid medication discontinuation and risk of adverse opioid-related health care events. *J Substance Abuse Treatm.* 2019;103:58–63.
69. Ballantyne JC, Sullivan MD, Koob GF. Refractory dependence on opioid analgesics. *Pain.* 2019;160(12):2655–2660.
70. Stumbo SP, Yarborough BJH, McCarty D, Weisner C, Green CA. Patient-reported pathways to opioid use disorders and pain-related barriers to treatment engagement. *J Substance Abuse Treatm.* 2017;73:47–54.
71. Mehl-Madrona L, Mainguy B, Plummer J. Integration of complementary and alternative medicine therapies into primary-care pain management for opiate reduction in a rural setting. *J Altern Complement Med.* 2016;22(8):621–626.
72. Sullivan M, Turner JA, DiLodovico C, D'Appollonio A, Stephens K, Chan Y-F. Prescription opioid taper support for outpatients with chronic pain: A randomized controlled trial. *J Pain.* 2017;18(3):308–318.
73. Zgierska AE, Burzinski CA, Cox J, et al. Mindfulness meditation and cognitive be-havioral therapy intervention reduces pain severity and sensitivity in opioid-treated chronic low back pain: Pilot findings from a randomized controlled trial. *Pain Med.* 2016;17(10):1865–1881.
74. Miller-Matero LR, Chohan S, Gavrilova L, et al. Utilizing primary care to engage patients on opioids in a psychological intervention for chronic pain. *Substance Use Misuse.* 2022;57(9):1492–1496.
75. Garland EL, Manusov EG, Froeliger B, Kelly A, Williams JM, Howard MO. Mindfulness-oriented recovery enhancement for chronic pain and prescription opioid misuse: Results from an early-stage randomized controlled trial. *J Consult Clin Psychol.* 2014;82(3):448.
76. Barry DT, Beitel M, Cutter CJ, et al. An evaluation of the feasibility, acceptability, and preliminary efficacy of cognitive-behavioral therapy for opioid use disorder and chronic pain. *Drug Alcohol Depend.* 2019;194:460–467.
77. Morley S, Eccleston C, Williams A. Systematic review and meta-analysis of randomized controlled trials of cognitive behaviour therapy and behaviour therapy for chronic pain in adults, excluding headache. *Pain.* 1999;80(1–2):1–13.
78. Dixon KE, Keefe FJ, Scipio CD, Perri LM, Abernethy APJHP. Psychological interventions for arthritis pain management in adults: A meta-analysis. *Health Psychol.* 2007;26(3):241.
79. Penney LS, Ritenbaugh C, DeBar LL, Elder C, Deyo RA. Provider and patient perspectives on opioids and alternative treatments for managing chronic pain: A qualitative study. *BMC Fam Pract.* 2016;17(1):1–15.
80. Becker WC, Dorflinger L, Edmond SN, Islam L, Heapy AA, Fraenkel L. Barriers and facilitators to use of non-pharmacological treatments in chronic pain. *BMC Fam Pract.* 2017;18(1):41.
81. Bair MJ, Matthias MS, Nyland KA, et al. Barriers and facilitators to chronic pain self-management: A qualitative study of primary care patients with comorbid musculoskeletal pain and depression. *Pain Med.* 2009;10(7):1280–1290.
82. Nicholas MK, Asghari A, Blyth FM, et al. Long-term outcomes from training in self-management of chronic pain in an elderly population: A randomized controlled trial. *Pain.* 2016;158(1):86–95.

83. Carmody TP. Psychosocial subgroups, coping, and chronic low-back pain. *J Clin Psychol Med Set*. 2001;8:137–148.
84. Davis M, Addis ME. Predictors of attrition from behavioral medicine treatments. *Ann Behav Med*. 1999;21(4):339–349.
85. Schappert SM. National Ambulatory Medical Care Survey: 1989 summary. Vital and health statistics Series 13, Data from the National Health Survey. *Vital Health Stat 13*. 1992(110):1–80.
86. Mäntyselkä P, Kumpusalo E, Ahonen R, et al. Pain as a reason to visit the doctor: A study in Finnish primary health care. *Pain*. 2001;89(2):175–180.
87. Miller-Matero LR, Dubaybo F, Ziadni MS, et al. Embedding a psychologist into primary care increases access to behavioral health services. *J Prim Care Comm Health*. 2015;6(2):100–104.
88. Guck TP, Guck AJ, Brack AB, Frey DR. No-show rates in partially integrated models of behavioral health care in a primary care setting. *Families Systems Health*. 2007;25(2):137.
89. Pomerantz A, Cole BH, Watts BV, Weeks WB. Improving efficiency and access to mental health care: Combining integrated care and advanced access. *Gen Hosp Psychiatry*. 2008;30(6):546–551.
90. Brawer PA, Martielli R, Pye PL, Manwaring J, Tierney A. St. Louis Initiative for Integrated Care Excellence (SLI²CE): Integrated-collaborative care on a large scale model. *Families Systems Health*. 2010;28(2):175.
91. Bohnert KM, Pfeiffer PN, Szymanski BR, McCarthy JF. Continuation of care following an initial primary care visit with a mental health diagnosis: Differences by receipt of VHA Primary Care–Mental Health Integration services. *Gen Hosp Psychiatry*. 2013;35(1):66–70.
92. Szymanski BR, Bohnert KM, Zivin K, McCarthy JF. Integrated care: Treatment initiation following positive depression screens. *J Gen Intern Med*. 2013;28(3):346–352.
93. Vickers KS, Ridgeway JL, Hathaway JC, Egginton JS, Kaderlik AB, Katzelnick DJ. Integration of mental health resources in a primary care setting leads to increased provider satisfaction and patient access. *Gen Hosp Psychiatry*. 2013;35(5):461–467.
94. Horevitz E, Organista KC, Arean PA. Depression treatment uptake in integrated primary care: How a "warm handoff" and other factors affect decision making by Latinos. *Psychiatric Serv*. 2015;66:824–830.
95. Reid RJ, Coleman K, Johnson EA, et al. The group health medical home at year two: Cost savings, higher patient satisfaction, and less burnout for providers. *Health Aff*. 2010;29(5):835–843.
96. Funderburk JS, Sugarman DE, Maisto SA, et al. The description and evaluation of the implementation of an integrated healthcare model. *Families Systems Health*. 2010;28(2):146.
97. Reiss-Brennan B. Mental health integration normalizing team care. *J Prim Care Comm Health*. 2013:2150131913508983.
98. Jackson GL, Powers BJ, Chatterjee R, et al. The patient-centered medical home: A systematic review. *Ann Intern Med*. 2013;158(3):169–178.
99. Schoen C, Osborn R, Squires D, Doty M, Pierson R, Applebaum S. New 2011 survey of patients with complex care needs in eleven countries finds that care is often poorly coordinated. *Health Aff*. 2011;30(12):2437–2448.
100. Miller-Matero LR, Dykuis KE, Albujoq K, et al. Benefits of integrated behavioral health services: The physician perspective. *Families Systems Health*. 2016;34(1):51.
101. Miller-Matero LR, Hecht L, Miller MK, et al. A brief psychological intervention for chronic pain in primary care: A pilot randomized controlled trial. *Pain Med*. 2021;22:1603–1611.
102. Miller-Matero LR, Gavrilova L, Hecht LM, et al. A brief psychological intervention for chronic pain in primary care: Examining long-term effects from a pilot randomized clinical trial. *Pain Pract*. 2022;22:564–570.

103. Herbert MS, Afari N, Liu L, et al. Telehealth versus in-person acceptance and commitment therapy for chronic pain: A randomized noninferiority trial. *J Pain*. 2017;18(2):200–211.
104. Parker SJ, Jessel S, Richardson JE, Reid MCJBg. Older adults are mobile too! Identifying the barriers and facilitators to older adults' use of mHealth for pain management. *BMC Geriatr*. 2013;13(1):43.
105. Tobin ET, Hadwiger A, DiChiara A, Entz A, Miller-Matero LR. Demographic predictors of telehealth use for integrated psychological services in primary care during the COVID-19 pandemic. *J Racial Ethnic Health Disparities*. 2023 Jun;10(3):1492–1498.
106. Chen I, Kurz J, Pasanen M, et al. Racial differences in opioid use for chronic nonmalignant pain. *J Gen Intern Med*. 2005;20(7):593–598.
107. Ringwalt C, Roberts AW, Gugelmann H, Skinner AC. Racial disparities across provider specialties in opioid prescriptions dispensed to Medicaid beneficiaries with chronic noncancer pain. *Pain Med*. 2015;16(4):633–640.
108. Morales ME, Yong RJ. Racial and ethnic disparities in the treatment of chronic pain. *Pain Med*. 2021;22(1):75–90.
109. Hausmann LR, Gao S, Lee ES, Kwoh CK. Racial disparities in the monitoring of patients on chronic opioid therapy. *Pain*. 2013;154(1):46–52.
110. Mossey JM. Defining racial and ethnic disparities in pain management. *Clin Orthopaed Related Res*. 2011;469(7):1859–1870.
111. Green CR, Baker TA, Sato Y, Washington TL, Smith EM. Race and chronic pain: A comparative study of young black and white Americans presenting for management. *J Pain*. 2003;4(4):176–183.
112. Dobalian A, Rivers PA. Racial and ethnic disparities in the use of mental health services. *J Behav Health Serv Res*. 2008;35(2):128–141.
113. US Surgeon General. *Mental Health: Culture, Race, and Ethnicity. A Supplement to Mental Health: A Report of the Surgeon General*. US Department of Health Human Services; 2001.
114. Padgett DK, Patrick C, Burns BJ, Schlesinger HJ. Ethnicity and the use of outpatient mental health services in a national insured population. *Am J Publ Health*. 1994;84(2):222–226.
115. Rintala A, Rantalainen R, Kaksonen A, Luomajoki H, Kauranen K. mHealth apps for low back pain self-management: scoping review. *JMIR mHealth uHealth*. 2022;10(8):e39682.
116. Pierik JG, IJzerman MJ, Gaakeer M, Vollenbroek-Hutten MMR, Vugt A, Doggen CJM. Incidence and prognostic factors of chronic pain after isolated musculoskeletal extremity injury. *Eur J Pain*. 2016;20(5):711–722.
117. Hasenbring M, Hallner D, Klasen B. Psychological mechanisms in the transition from acute to chronic pain: over-or underrated? *Schmerz (Berlin, Germany)*. 2001;15(6):442–447.
118. Casey CY, Greenberg MA, Nicassio PM, Harpin RE, Hubbard D. Transition from acute to chronic pain and disability: A model including cognitive, affective, and trauma factors. *Pain*. 2008;134(1):69–79.
119. Vranceanu A-M, Bachoura A, Weening A, Vrahas M, Smith RM, Ring D. Psychological factors predict disability and pain intensity after skeletal trauma. *JBJS*. 2014;96(3):e20.
120. McLean SA, Clauw DJ, Abelson JL, Liberzon I. The development of persistent pain and psychological morbidity after motor vehicle collision: integrating the potential role of stress response systems into a biopsychosocial model. *Psychosomatic med*. 2005;67(5):783–790.
121. Helmerhorst GT, Vranceanu A-M, Vrahas M, Smith M, Ring D. Risk factors for continued opioid use one to two months after surgery for musculoskeletal trauma. *JBJS*. 2014;96(6):495–499.

DEPRESSION AND PAIN 79

122. Rozet I, Nishio I, Robbertze R, Rotter D, Chansky H, Hernandez AV. Prolonged opioid use after knee arthroscopy in military veterans. *Anesth Analg.* 2014;119(2):454–459.

123. Berge DJ, Dolin SJ, Williams AC, Harman R. Pre-operative and post-operative effect of a pain management programme prior to total hip replacement: A randomized controlled trial. *Pain.* 2004;110(1–2):33–39.

124. Dowsey M, Castle D, Knowles S, et al. The effect of mindfulness training prior to total joint arthroplasty on post-operative pain and physical function: A randomised controlled trial. *Complement Ther Med.* 2019;46:195–201.

125. Miller-Matero LR, Coleman JP, Smith-Mason CE, Moore DA, Marszalek D, Ahmedani BK. A brief mindfulness intervention for medically hospitalized patients with acute pain: A pilot randomized clinical trial. *Pain Med.* 2019;20:2149–2154.

126. Kathol RG, Butler M, McAlpine DD, Kane RL. Barriers to physical and mental condition integrated service delivery. *Psychosomatic Med.* 2010;72(6):511–518.

127. Cummings NA, O'Donohue WT, Cummings JL. The financial dimension of integrated behavioral/primary care. *J Clin Psychol Med Set.* 2009;16(1):31–39.

128. Kessler R, Stafford D, Messier R. The problem of integrating behavioral health in the medical home and the questions it leads to. *J Clin Psychol Med Set.* 2009;16(1):4–12.

129. Robinson P, Reiter J. *Behavioral Consultation and Primary Care.* Springer; 2007.

130. Gunn WB, Blount A. Primary care mental health: A new frontier for psychology. *J Clin Psychol.* 2009;65(3):235–252.

131. Klein S, Hostetter M. In focus: Integrating behavioral health and primary care. *Quality matters: Innovations in health care quality improvement.* 2014. https://www.commo nwealthfund.org/publications/newsletter-article/2014/aug/focus-integrating-behavio ral-health-and-primary-care

6

Other Psychiatric Disorders, Psychosocial Factors, Sleep, and Pain

Matthew J. Bair and Ashli A. Owen-Smith

6.1 Introduction

Chronic pain is frequently comorbid with psychiatric disorders.[1-3] While depression has been the most extensively studied comorbid psychiatric disorder in people with chronic pain,[4] there has been growing research on the high rates of comorbidity between chronic pain and anxiety disorders,[1,2] posttraumatic stress disorder (PTSD),[3] bipolar disorder (BD),[5] and schizophrenia.[6]

After depression, anxiety disorders are the most frequently studied comorbidity with chronic pain.[7] Chronic pain and anxiety commonly co-occur,[2] and this comorbidity is associated with worse outcomes than either chronic pain or anxiety alone. Anxiety disorders are the most frequently diagnosed psychiatric disorders overall[8] and represent a heterogenous family of conditions which include specific phobias, social anxiety disorder, panic disorder, agoraphobia, and generalized anxiety disorder. Approximately 30% of U.S. adults experience an anxiety disorder during their lifetime,[9] and at least 50% experience multiple anxiety disorders concomitantly. Anxiety disorders are frequently comorbid with mood and substance use disorders.[10] Notably, the presence of an anxiety disorder increases the risk of developing depression more than any other clinical factor.[11]

The prevalence of anxiety disorders in people with chronic pain is at least 25%,[12] yet the prevalence varies significantly[13] depending on (1) methods used to assess anxiety (structured diagnostic criteria or self-reported symptoms), (2) assessment time window (current disorder or lifetime), (3) sample type (general population, community-based, or clinical sample), (4) study setting (primary care, pain clinic, or mental health setting), and (5) spectrum of anxiety disorders and pain conditions studied. Multiple studies have evaluated the prevalence of psychiatric disorders in pain

Matthew J. Bair and Ashli A. Owen-Smith, *Other Psychiatric Disorders, Psychosocial Factors, Sleep, and Pain* In: *Pain, the Opioid Epidemic, & Depression*. Edited by: Jeffrey F. Scherrer & Jane C. Ballantyne, Oxford University Press. © Oxford University Press 2024. DOI: 10.1093/9780197675250.003.0006

samples[2,14-16] while relatively fewer studies have assessed the prevalence of chronic pain in clinical populations with psychiatric disorders.[6,17,18]

Psychiatric disorders are associated with the overall experience and perception of pain.[19] Comorbid psychiatric disorders are associated with worse pain and pain-related outcomes.[20] For example, anxiety is associated with greater pain intensity and pain interference in people with chronic pain[21] relative to those without anxiety. Conversely, chronic pain adversely affects mental health outcomes (e.g., symptom severity) in patients with psychiatric disorders.[22] Chronic pain has been found to reduce the effectiveness of antidepressant treatment and to decrease quality of life[23] in primary care patients being treated with selective serotonin reuptake inhibitors (SSRIs) for depression. Psychiatric disorders often co-occur with chronic low back pain.[14] Yet the strength of associations between psychiatric disorders and different chronic pain conditions may vary and be greater for painful conditions such as fibromyalgia,[24] irritable bowel syndrome,[25] and migraine headaches.[26]

Evidence suggests that sleep problems are common among patients with chronic pain, with up to 89% of patients reporting at least one sleep complaint and 53% of patients attending pain clinics presenting with clinically significant insomnia.[27,28] Indeed, severe pain is the most common cause of poor sleep,[29] and poor sleep may be further exacerbated for patients with chronic pain prescribed opioids because sleep disturbance is a common side effect.[30] The co-occurrence of sleep problems and chronic pain coupled with psychiatric disorders further diminishes quality of life; evidence suggests that individuals with psychiatric illnesses and comorbid sleep problems have increased risk of chronic pain compared to those without psychiatric illnesses,[31] and individuals with psychiatric conditions and comorbid chronic pain have increased risk of poor sleep quality.[32] Thus, the well-established and bidirectional relationship between poor sleep and chronic pain[33] may have particularly important implications for individuals with psychiatric conditions.

6.2 Chronic Pain and Anxiety

6.2.1 Epidemiology

Several epidemiological studies show that chronic pain and anxiety frequently co-occur. An international study of more than 85,000 community-living adults found those with back or neck pain had two to three times the likelihood of panic disorder, agoraphobia, or social anxiety disorder and three times the likelihood of generalized anxiety disorder.[34] A population-based study in Israel found an adjusted odds ratio (OR) of 2.94 (95% confidence interval [CI]: 2.08, 4.17) for anxiety disorders in people with chronic pain.[35] In the U.S. National Comorbidity Survey Part II, anxiety disorders, as assessed by *Diagnostic Statistical Manual of Mental Disorders III Revised* (DSM-III R) were present in 35% of a community-based sample with chronic arthritis pain compared to 17% of the general population.[36] A follow-up study of the National Comorbidity Survey examined respondents with chronic pain and showed that 26.5% had an anxiety disorder,[37] which translated to approximately 10.5 million U.S. adults with comorbid chronic pain and anxiety disorders. Individuals with comorbid chronic pain and sleep disturbance may have an even greater risk for anxiety-related symptoms, and anxiety has been reported to be a risk factor associated with sleep disturbances in patients with chronic pain.[38]

Studies of comorbidity in clinical settings have typically examined the prevalence of significant anxiety symptoms or anxiety disorders in patients with chronic pain.[39] Overall, the prevalence of anxiety in clinical samples ranges between 20% and 30%.[40,41] However, prevalence varies depending on study setting and on whether a structured clinical interview or self-reported symptom measure was used to assess anxiety.[42] Another factor that affects prevalence is whether current disorder or lifetime anxiety disorders are assessed. Atkinson et al.[14] found relatively high rates of generalized anxiety, panic disorder, and obsessive-compulsive disorders in patients with pain. A more recent study by Knaster and colleagues[2] found that the prevalence of anxiety disorders, based on a structured diagnostic interview, was 25% in patients referred to a pain clinic. In pain clinic samples, panic disorder and generalized anxiety disorder are the most diagnosed anxiety disorders.[34,43,44] In primary care, 45% of patients with chronic pain screened positive for one or more anxiety disorders.[45] Women with chronic pelvic pain had twice the prevalence of anxiety (73% vs. 37%) as those without chronic pelvic pain.[46] Relatively few studies have examined the prevalence of chronic pain in samples with anxiety disorders. In one study, of patients referred to a mental health clinic for panic disorder, 40% reported chronic pain, mainly of musculoskeletal origin.[47] Of note, all these studies were published when the DSM-IV classified PTSD as an anxiety disorder.

Comorbidity studies raise the question of which condition develops first, anxiety or chronic pain. Kinney et al.[48] found 23% of patients with chronic

OTHER PSYCHIATRIC DISORDERS   83

low back pain had a preexisting anxiety disorder. In a Finnish pain clinic, Knaster et al.[2] found that most anxiety disorders (77%) were present before pain developed. In another study, more than 50% of people developed an anxiety disorder after the onset of chronic pain.[14] These studies do not provide convincing evidence of which condition is more likely to develop first, however they strongly suggest a bidirectional relationship between chronic pain and anxiety disorders.[39]

Anxiety disorders, especially panic disorder and generalized anxiety disorder, and chronic pain share several psychological vulnerabilities[39] which likely explains their frequent overlap. These vulnerabilities include hyperarousal, somatic cues, and attentional biases, which can underlie pain and anxiety.[49] The relationship between chronic pain and anxiety disorders may depend on the specific pain condition studied. In patients with chronic low back pain, 31% met criteria for at least one current psychiatric disorder as assessed by diagnostic interview,[16] with anxiety disorders present in 12% of patients. Almost one-third of patients with fibromyalgia had a current or lifetime panic disorder or PTSD.[24] Women with fibromyalgia compared to those without fibromyalgia were four to five times more likely to have a lifetime diagnosis of obsessive-compulsive disorder, PTSD, or generalized anxiety disorder.[44] Patients with irritable bowel syndrome have threefold increased odds of either anxiety or depression, compared to healthy participants.[50] In primary care, the likelihood of anxiety increases with the number of painful symptoms reported.[51] In another primary care study, patients who reported muscle pain, headache, or stomach pain were 2.5–10 times more likely to screen positive for panic disorder, generalized anxiety disorder, or major depressive disorder.[52]

6.2.2 Impact of Comorbid Chronic Pain and Anxiety on Clinical Outcomes

Comorbid chronic pain and anxiety add clinical complexity, negatively affect outcomes, and cause more morbidity and disability than either condition alone. A classic experimental pain study[53] showed that anxiety leads to increased pain reactivity and lower heat pain thresholds suggesting a lower tolerance to pain. Several studies have linked anxiety symptoms and anxiety disorders to outcomes in patients with chronic pain. Psychological distress, particularly depression and anxiety, are the most common risk factors for

84 MATTHEW J. BAIR AND ASHLI A. OWEN-SMITH

back pain in young people,[54] and anxiety is associated with more frequent pain episodes.[55] Furthermore, anxiety is associated with increased pain intensity, greater pain interference,[21] more pain-related disability, longer duration of pain, and poorer response to treatment. Anxiety can negatively affect adaptive thoughts, coping, and self-care behaviors which may hinder rehabilitation, thus increasing the risk of pain-related disability.[56]

More severe pain is associated with a higher risk for developing incident anxiety[57] and more severe anxiety symptoms.[58] Primary care patients with chronic pain who screen positive for anxiety disorders have significantly worse health-related quality of life, especially worse mental health functioning.[45] Furthermore, patients progressively worsened as the number of concomitant anxiety disorders increased, leading to even greater pain interference and more disability days related to pain.[45] These findings strongly suggest that chronic pain makes functioning across several areas even more difficult for those individuals with a concomitant anxiety disorder.

6.2.3 Clinical Assessment in Comorbid Chronic Pain and Anxiety

Due to the frequent comorbidity between chronic pain and psychiatric disorders, clinical practice guidelines recommend conducting a comprehensive assessment of pain and concomitant psychiatric disorders in all patients with chronic pain.[59,60] Screening patients with chronic pain for psychiatric conditions, especially anxiety, is important since comorbid anxiety can negatively impact outcomes[61,62] and lead to greater healthcare utilization.[63]

The biopsychosocial model[64] is a useful framework and guide to the clinical assessment and symptom monitoring in patients with chronic pain and anxiety. Furthermore, the model can help elucidate the interplay between biological, psychological, and social factors that underlie the potential causes and development of chronic pain and anxiety comorbidity. Several pain and anxiety measures can be administered across biopsychosocial domains to achieve a comprehensive assessment, establish an accurate diagnosis, and facilitate patient–clinician discussions about effective treatments that address relevant biopsychosocial domains in the context of chronic pain and anxiety comorbidity.

In busy clinical practices, administering a set of brief measures is an efficient method to assess pain and all of its different facets, including functional status and common psychological comorbidities. The National Institute of Health's (NIH) Pain Consortium offers guidance on specific measures that can be used for screening and monitoring pain and anxiety. The NIH Pain Consortium has compiled a useful resource library for clinicians called "Pain Assessment Resources for Professionals" that includes several pain and pain-related questionnaires at https://www.painconsortium.nih.gov/resou rce-library/resources-pain-assessment. For pain assessment, this resource library highlights Patient-Reported Outcomes Measurement Information System (PROMIS) measures (https://commonfund.nih.gov/promis/index) to assess multiple pain-relevant domains (pain intensity, pain interference, pain quality, pain behaviors, physical function, self-efficacy, fatigue, sleep quality) and the brief (three-item) PEG-3 to assess pain intensity and pain interference.[65]

Anxiety disorders frequently go unrecognized in primary care[66,67] and pain care settings[68] because symptoms are often attributed to physical causes, such as pain, rather than psychological conditions. The focus on pain can obscure the clinician and patient's awareness that an anxiety disorder is also present. Other barriers to recognizing anxiety disorders include time constraints and competing priorities in clinical practice. When anxiety disorders are unrecognized they frequently go untreated[67] which adversely affects patients with anxiety and can lead to suboptimal pain management.

To aid in anxiety disorder diagnosis and assessment of anxiety symptoms, the GAD-2 is an ultra-brief, two-item, screening tool that asks about the frequency of anxiety or uncontrollable worry over the past 2 weeks.[69] If a patient screens positive, a more comprehensive measure such as the GAD-7,[70] Hospital Anxiety and Depression Scale (HADS),[71] or the Spielberger State Trait Anxiety Inventory can be used to assess anxiety symptom severity. If symptoms are moderate to severe, it may be clinically indicated to refer to a mental health clinician. Another relevant measure in patients with chronic pain and anxiety is the Pain Anxiety Symptoms Scale which measures behavioral responses (e.g., complaining, withdrawing from activities) to pain.[72] Because distinguishing between anxiety disorders is difficult and there are common overlaps between anxiety and other psychiatric disorders, a structured diagnostic interview by a trained mental health clinician is considered the gold standard to diagnose specific anxiety disorders according to DSM-5 criteria.

6.2.4 Pharmacological Treatment of Comorbid Chronic Pain and Anxiety

Clinical practice guidelines regarding the pharmacological treatment for chronic pain[73] or for the treatment of anxiety disorders[74,75] have been published. These guidelines provide an in-depth discussion and guidance on pharmacological treatment which readers can refer to. Several medications are effective in treating anxiety disorders[76,77] and include serotonin-norepinephrine reuptake inhibitors (SNRIs), SSRIs, tricyclic antidepressants (TCAs), azapirones (e.g., buspirone), mixed antidepressants (e.g., mirtazapine), antipsychotics, antihistamines (e.g., hydroxyzine), and benzodiazepines. Although benzodiazepines are not recommended for routine use,[78] they can be helpful in the short term and for acute anxiety.

While SSRIs are commonly used for anxiety disorders, their effectiveness in chronic pain conditions has been inconsistent[79,80] and, when shown to be effective, generally provide minimal pain relief. Experts opine that non-opioid medications, such as SNRIs, TCAs, and anticonvulsants, have a role in the multimodal treatment of patients with chronic pain and anxiety by relieving symptoms[81] due to their dual effects on relieving pain and anxiety. These medications are often referred to as *co-analgesics* or *adjuvant pain medications* because their initial development and primary clinical indication was for non-pain conditions such as depression, anxiety, or seizure disorders. Yet with clinical experience and in subsequent clinical trials these medications have provided pain relief for some individuals.

The SNRIs (duloxetine, venlafaxine, and milnacipran) and the TCAs (amitriptyline, nortriptyline, and desipramine) can lessen neuropathic pain severity[82,83] and headache frequency.[84] A recent review[85] found moderate certainty evidence for SNRIs for back pain, postoperative pain, neuropathic pain, and fibromyalgia. Duloxetine can ease pain in patients with diabetic peripheral neuropathy,[86-88] fibromyalgia,[89] and chronic low back pain—three chronic pain conditions with frequent psychiatric comorbidity. Venlafaxine, another SNRI, has been used to treat neuropathic pain, fibromyalgia, and tension headaches but evidence for its effectiveness is weak.[90] TCAs, when used to treat neuropathic pain, are prescribed at lower doses than when used primarily for anxiety. The anticonvulsants, especially gabapentin and pregabalin, have been used for anxiety[91] and for treatment of neuropathic and central pain conditions.[92] For example, pregabalin is approved by the

U.S. Food and Drug Administration (FDA) for diabetic peripheral neuropathy, postherpetic neuralgia, and fibromyalgia.

Nonsteroidal anti-inflammatory drugs (NSAIDs) and acetaminophen are simple analgesics frequently used to treat acute and chronic pain but do not have any direct anxiolytic effects. Their renal, gastrointestinal, and cardiovascular side effects are well-known,[93] particularly in older adults.[94] In treating patients with chronic pain and anxiety, it is important to be aware of potential drug-drug interactions. Individually, NSAIDs or SSRIs increase the risk of gastrointestinal bleeding when used long-term so using them in combination may further increase the risk of bleeding.[95] The concomitant use of tramadol and SSRIs is associated with serotonin syndrome and can decrease an individual's seizure threshold. Although lithium is typically used for BD and not anxiety disorders, NSAIDs can increase blood lithium levels,[96] potentially leading to side effects such as confusion, tremor, slurred speech, and vomiting. Acetaminophen and SSRIs are metabolized in the liver by some of the same cytochrome P450 enzymes, which may lead to interactions and require more frequent monitoring of liver enzyme tests.

6.2.5 Opioid Therapy in the Context of Comorbid Pain and Anxiety

A systematic review[97] found that people with anxiety and/or depression are significantly more likely to develop problematic opioid use when treated with opioids for chronic pain[97] than individuals without anxiety and/or depression. Therefore, frequent monitoring of opioid use, opioid-related problems (abuse, misuse), and side effect management (constipation, sedation, nausea, pruritus, and urinary retention) are warranted in patients with chronic pain and anxiety. Psychological support in the context of comorbid chronic pain and anxiety is critical. While benzodiazepines are occasionally used for anxiety disorders, prescribing a benzodiazepine and an opioid concurrently is generally discouraged due to their potential interactions and the additive risk for respiratory depression and overdose.[98] Other medication interactions to consider are concomitant use of codeine or hydrocodone with paroxetine, bupropion, and duloxetine. Because these medications compete for the same liver enzyme (CYP-2D6), the analgesic effects of codeine and hydrocodone may be lessened.[99]

6.2.6 Non-Pharmacological Management of Comorbid Chronic Pain and Anxiety

While educational programs alone are insufficient to significantly improve pain outcomes,[100] education is foundational and can help patients better understand their pain and how anxiety may influence their pain. Providing education can help clinicians build rapport with their patients, create a therapeutic alliance, and offer rationale for treatment decisions. Furthermore, educational programs often introduce and discuss self-management strategies (physical activity, goal setting, pacing activities) and lifestyle changes (stress management, adequate sleep, healthy diet) which can improve pain and anxiety symptoms. As a result, education has an essential role in the non-pharmacological management of chronic pain and anxiety.

Several psychological and behavioral interventions (e.g., cognitive behavioral therapy [CBT], acceptance and commitment therapy, coping skills training, relaxation training, hypnosis, exercise, and mindfulness-based stress reduction) have been used and tested in patients with chronic pain or anxiety individually. These therapies can be used on their own to treat pain in patients with anxiety or as adjuncts to medication treatment. CBT is the most extensively studied psychological treatment for chronic pain[101] or anxiety disorders,[102] and underlying CBT principles can be applied to chronic pain and anxiety comorbidity. For a more comprehensive discussion, please refer to Chapter 5, devoted to psychological therapies for comorbid pain and depression.

6.3 Chronic Pain and Posttraumatic Stress Disorder

6.3.1 Epidemiology

PTSD and chronic pain frequently coexist because their development is preceded by traumatic experiences. Yet the prevalence of this comorbidity depends on factors such as study setting, sample characteristics, and how PTSD symptoms are assessed or if diagnostic criteria are used and met. Two separate studies in multidisciplinary pain clinic samples revealed that almost 30% of patients had PTSD symptoms.[103,104] In patients with traumatic pain after a motor vehicle accident, 30–50% reported symptoms of PTSD.[105] Among injured workers, PTSD was present in 35%,[106] and more than 45%

OTHER PSYCHIATRIC DISORDERS 89

of patients with fibromyalgia compared to 3% of population-based controls met criteria for PTSD.[107]

The prevalence of chronic pain in persons with a PTSD diagnosis is high. Pain is the most common physical symptom in patients with PTSD.[108] Among 340 Operation Iraqi Freedom/Operation Enduring Freedom veterans included in a polytrauma network registry, 42% had medical record-confirmed comorbid chronic pain, PTSD, and persistent postconcussive symptoms.[109] In patients seeking treatment for PTSD from community-based mental health clinics, approximately 30% reported chronic pain,[110] and upward of 60–80% of military veterans with PTSD have chronic pain.[3,111,112]

Häuser and colleagues assessed the bidirectional nature of pain and PTSD and showed that PTSD symptoms preceded the onset of chronic widespread pain in 66.5% of patients,[107] while PTSD symptoms followed the onset of chronic widespread pain in 29.5%. PTSD is a potential risk factor for fibromyalgia and vice versa.[107] In the National Comorbidity Survey, Part II, significant positive associations were found between chronic pain and mood and anxiety disorders (OR ranged from 1.92 to 4.27). After panic disorder (OR = 4.27), the strongest association was observed for PTSD (OR = 3.69).[113]

Sleep disturbance is one potentially modifiable mechanism that may underlie the co-occurrence of chronic pain and PTSD.[114] Insomnia occurs in 60–90% of patients with PTSD.[115] PTSD symptom severity has also been associated with insomnia and pain severity in a veteran sample.[116] This mechanism may be explained in part by the ways in which hyperarousal (a classic PTSD symptom) may result in difficulty falling or staying asleep and impairment in overall sleep quality resulting in increased pain sensitivity, pain-related anxiety, and pain-avoidant behaviors, which in turn can result in chronic pain. Ongoing sleep disturbances may serve to maintain PTSD and chronic pain over time. For example, one study[114] reported that, even after controlling for associated demographic characteristics, higher levels of PTSD symptoms were linked to higher levels of pain intensity and pain interference, and these relationships were partially explained by poor sleep quality.[114] Another study similarly reported that veterans with PTSD and pain demonstrated greater sleep disturbance compared to veterans without PTSD.[117] Mental health comorbidities coupled with the high prevalence of chronic pain escalates veterans' risk for opioid misuse and abuse[118] that further contribute to sleep disturbances and sleep disorders.[119]

6.3.2 Impact of Comorbid Chronic Pain and Posttraumatic Stress Disorder on Clinical Outcomes

When chronic pain and PTSD co-occur, the negative effects can be widespread and significantly worse than with either condition alone. Both community and veteran samples have demonstrated the negative impacts of pain–PTSD comorbidity on prognosis and treatment outcomes[120] and on several clinical and functional domains including psychological distress and pain severity,[121–123] psychosocial and physical impairment,[122,124] pain interference,[123] disability,[120,123] and quality of life.[125] PTSD can heighten pain severity, which may increase disability, and pain can worsen avoidance, a cardinal symptom of PTSD. Therefore, PTSD and pain can mutually reinforce and maintain each other unless effective treatment is delivered.[126]

Moreover, patients with chronic pain and PTSD comorbidity tend to employ ineffective coping strategies (fear avoidance) and often have maladaptive cognitions, such as catastrophizing thoughts, lower sense of control over pain, higher pain centrality, and lower perceived life control.[123,127,128] Patients with this co-occurrence report an increased risk of suicidal ideation compared to individuals experiencing chronic pain or PTSD alone.[129] Last, both conditions are associated with persistent disability, strongly influenced by social and emotional factors, and a lengthy, chronic course.[130] Studies suggest a "synergistic negative impact"[131] of chronic pain and PTSD comorbidity and argue for effective, concomitant treatment for both conditions.

6.3.3 Clinical Assessment of Comorbid Chronic Pain and Posttraumatic Stress Disorder

Detecting and treating PTSD is an important component of effective pain management. Clinical assessment of chronic pain and PTSD comorbidity is best guided by a biopsychosocial history conducted by treating clinicians. This biopsychosocial model for assessment helps clinicians better understand the interactions among biological, psychological, and social factors and then direct treatment to these factors. While the gold standard for PTSD assessment is the Clinician Administered PTSD Scale for DSM-5 (CAPS-5),[132] several briefer measures can be incorporated into clinical practice. One brief measure is the PTSD checklist for DSM-5 (PCL-5)[133] that can be used as a screening tool or to monitor PTSD symptoms longitudinally.[134] If patients screen positive for PTSD and exhibit moderate to severe PTSD symptoms, referral to a mental health clinician is appropriate for a comprehensive evaluation and discussion of various treatment options.

6.3.4 Pharmacological Management of Comorbid Pain and PTSD

Although not considered first-line treatment, pharmacological management can help alleviate PTSD symptoms.[135] For patients who prefer medications or who do not have access to trauma-focused psychotherapy, pharmacological management can be an effective option. PTSD is frequently comorbid with other psychiatric comorbidities (e.g., anxiety, depression) which are often treated with anxiolytics, antidepressants, mood stabilizers, or antipsychotics that influence the neurotransmitters involved in the fear and anxiety circuitry of the brain. A network meta-analysis[136] showed that paroxetine, venlafaxine, and quetiapine are considered first-line pharmacological treatments for PTSD. Additionally, quetiapine is recommended for symptoms of hyperarousal and re-experiencing of trauma in patients with PTSD.[136] Studies of pharmacological treatments for PTSD-related sleep disturbances are limited due to small sample sizes and other methodological flaws. Prazosin, an alpha-adrenergic receptor antagonist, has the strongest evidence for PTSD-related sleep disturbances, especially for nightmares.[137] The Standards of Practice Committee of the American Academy of Sleep Medicine[138] provides recommendations for prazosin and other agents (SSRIs, SNRIs, TCAs, atypical antipsychotics, benzodiazepines, sedative hypnotics, and anticonvulsants) for treating PTSD-associated nightmares.

6.3.5 Opioid Therapy in the Context of Comorbid Pain and Posttraumatic Stress Disorder

Seal and colleagues found receipt of prescription opioids was associated with more than twice the risk (9.5% vs. 4.1%) for adverse outcomes for veterans with mental health disorders,[139] particularly in veterans with PTSD. Veterans with PTSD who were prescribed opioids were more likely to receive higher-dose opioids (22.7% vs. 15.9%, adjusted relative risk [RR], 1.42; 95% CI: 1.31, 1.54) relative to those without mental health disorders, receive two or more opioids concurrently (19.8% vs. 10.7%, adjusted RR, 1.87; 95% CI: 1.70, 2.06), receive sedative hypnotics concurrently (40.7% vs. 7.6%, adjusted RR, 5.46; 95% CI: 4.91, 6.07), or obtain early opioid refills (33.8% vs. 20.4%; adjusted RR, 1.64; 95% CI: 1.53, 1.75).

In a retrospective cohort study of veterans with chronic pain, PTSD, and substance use disorders,[140] two cohorts were compared on longitudinal changes in PTSD symptoms. Almost a quarter (23.7%) of veterans in the buprenorphine/naloxone cohort versus 11.7% in the traditional opioid cohort showed improved PTSD symptoms (p = .001). The improvement in PTSD symptoms was modest but seen after 8 months and sustained at 24 months. Pain severity did not increase over time and there were no differences between groups. This study provides interesting observational data about the potential use of buprenorphine/naloxone in the integrated treatment of pain, PTSD, and substance use disorders but needs to be tested in a clinical trial.

6.3.6 Non-Pharmacological Management of Comorbid Chronic Pain and Posttraumatic Stress Disorder

As in chronic pain management, non-pharmacological interventions are recommended as first-line treatment for PTSD. Of the various trauma-focused psychotherapies, prolonged exposure (PE) and cognitive processing therapy (CPT) have the strongest evidence for PTSD treatment.[141] Clinical practice guidelines[142] also recommend other psychotherapies for PTSD treatment such as trauma-focused CBT and eye movement desensitization and reprocessing (EMDR).

CBT strategies (relaxation, pacing, activity scheduling, distraction, cognitive restructuring) can help patients understand how traumatic events experienced are related to their chronic pain and PTSD and can reduce pain scores, improve pain-related function, and relieve PTSD symptoms.[143-145] These strategies can also help reduce the hypervigilance and catastrophizing common in patients with chronic pain and PTSD.

However, the literature on treatment of comorbid chronic pain and PTSD is limited.

6.4 Chronic Pain and Bipolar Disorder

6.4.1 Epidemiology

Current research on pain conditions among individuals with BD consistently indicates that these individuals experience significant levels of pain. For example, a meta-analysis of prevalence studies found that the overall pooled analysis of pain in people with BD was 28.9% and the relative risk was more than doubled for people with BD compared to the general population.[5] In a cross-sectional study of the associations between pain and schizophrenia, depression, and BD among Veterans Health Affairs patients, Birgenheir et al.[6] observed that pain conditions were most common among those with depression followed by BD and least common in schizophrenia. In contrast, in analyses of more than 149,000 patients in the United Kingdom, Biobank revealed chronic pain was most prevalent (54.8%) among those with bipolar I and II, followed by depression (50.4%) and controls (38.2%).[146] This study also observed increasing prevalence of BD as the number of pain sites increased.[146] Owen-Smith and colleagues'[147] analysis of multiple, large private-sector healthcare systems in the United States revealed that, as compared to patients without a mental health diagnosis, there was a 71% greater risk for a pain diagnosis among those with BD. Others have observed nearly a fivefold increased risk for chronic pain in BD compared to controls.[148] Although there is variation in whether pain is more common in major depression, BD, or schizophrenia, most evidence indicates those with BD have a markedly higher risk for pain compared to persons without mental illness.

There is evidence that migraine is a unique burden for patients with BD. Migraine headache is twice as common among those with BD compared to the general population, and it is associated with worse outcomes.[149] Results from the Canadian Community Health Survey of more than 36,000 participants revealed that males with BD and comorbid migraine versus BD alone were more likely to have low income, require social assistance and welfare, have earlier age onset of BD, have high lifetime comorbid anxiety, and use more mental and physical healthcare.[149] Women with comorbid BD and migraine compared to BD alone required more personal and instrumental support in activities of daily living.[149] Oedegaard and Fasmer[150] suggest migraine headaches are a BD trait because the clinical characteristics of comorbid migraine and depression resemble some BD symptoms such as high rates of irritability and affective temperaments. Additional research is needed to determine the type of pain and pain locations that might distinguish comorbid pain in BD from pain comorbid in depression and schizophrenia.

One noteworthy risk factor for chronic pain among individuals with BD is the presence of sleep disorders.[151] Though the association between chronic pain and sleep difficulties is well-established in both psychiatric populations[33] and healthy controls,[152] it may be particularly problematic for individuals with BD since sleep disruption is the most common prodrome of mania.[153]

6.4.2 Impact of Comorbid Chronic Pain and Bipolar Disorder on Clinical Outcomes

Compared to those without serious mental illness, people with BD are more likely to experience conditions that cause pain,[154] and pain is also associated with worse psychiatric symptoms.[155] Evidence suggests that the presence of chronic pain for those with BD is associated with impaired recovery, greater functional incapacitation, lower quality of life, and increased risk of suicide compared to people without pain.[6,149,156-158] Comorbid pain in BD is associated with moderate to severe pain interference (the degree to which pain impairs activities of daily living) and worse mental health and BD related functioning.[159]

Interestingly, a qualitative study revealed that, for some patients with BD, pain appears to be less severe during manic or euphoric states while worsening during periods of irritability or anger[160]; this finding is consistent with a subsequent retrospective medical record analysis that similarly found that more than 64% of patients with chronic pain and comorbid BD reported experiencing reduced pain intensity during manic or hypomanic episodes. This may ultimately exacerbate their pain conditions if, during manic periods, they engage in more activity than recommended; this overexertion may worsen their pain conditions and/or make pain more noticeable when the mania phase resolves.[161] Patients also reported feeling disconnected from pain,[160] which is consistent with evidence of abnormal pain processing in patients with BD.[162]

6.4.3 Pharmacological Management for Comorbid Chronic Pain and Bipolar Disorder

There is significant overlap in the pharmacologic treatment of chronic pain and psychiatric disorders, including BD. For example, some third-generation antiepileptic medications used for patients with BD (as an alternative to lithium) and anticonvulsants (e.g., pregabalin or gabapentin) have also been used to treat certain chronic pain conditions (e.g., fibromyalgia, neuropathy, migraine, low back pain).[163,164] Chronic pain, especially neuropathic pain, is sometimes managed with TCAs; however, these medications for people with BD can trigger a manic episode if prescribed in the absence of a mood stabilizer.[165,166] Thus, there are unique considerations for the pharmacological treatment of chronic pain in individuals with BD. Furthermore, meta-analyses suggest that only approximately half of patients experience clinically meaningful improvements in pain from pharmacological therapies,[167-170] and many individuals discontinue these medications due to negative side effects or lack of efficacy.[171]

Cannabis is increasingly legal for treating chronic pain, among other medical conditions. Evidence about cannabis in pain management—particularly for chronic neuropathic pain—is conflicting: though one review paper reported cannabinoids as "modestly effective,"[172] others have found no high-quality evidence of efficacy; thus, cannabis has only been recommended in several consensus guidelines as a third- or fourth-line treatment for pain.[173,174] Of note, however, is that cannabis use was associated with the development of BD in an analysis of National Epidemiologic Survey on Alcohol and Related Conditions data.[175] Furthermore, a recent overview of systematic reviews reported risks related to cannabis use specific to those with BD, including an increased risk of mania, greater symptom severity, greater number of symptoms, and less frequent remission from mania and depression.[176] Thus, cannabis use for pain may be particularly risky, especially for those at greater risk of BD.

6.4.4 Opioid Therapy in the Context of Comorbid Chronic Pain and Bipolar Disorder

Evidence suggests that individuals with BD are significantly more likely to receive long-term opioids, at a higher daily dose, and with greater days supplied compared with patients without mental illness[147,177-182] despite evidence that persons with mental illness may benefit less from opioid therapy compared to individuals without psychiatric morbidities.[183] One explanation for this is that these individuals may present with greater pain severity and worse physical functioning, thereby increasing the likelihood that clinicians will prescribe an opioid and at a higher dose.[184] Ironically, prior studies have reported diminished opioid analgesia for individuals with psychiatric diagnoses[183]; thus, these medications are likely to be less effective for pain management.

Potential risks are associated with medical and non-medical opioid use specifically for individuals with BD. Several case studies have reported significant hypomanic/manic reactions,[185,186] antidepressant effects,[185] and psychotic symptoms[187] following opioid use in this population. Conversely, the incidence and prevalence of BD and related symptoms increase after the initiation of opioid use or during long-term opioid use.[188] For example, Schepis and colleagues[189] compared the prevalence of BD at follow-up between people who engaged in weekly or daily use of nonmedical prescription opioids and people who used opioids monthly or less frequently. They found that weekly/daily use predicted higher odds of BD.[189] Finally, prior studies have reported that having a history of BD may place these individuals at an increased risk for non-medical opioid dependence.[190-192]

6.4.5 Non-Pharmacological Management of Comorbid Chronic Pain and Bipolar Disorder

CBT for chronic pain is a non-pharmacological treatment that aims to reduce pain perception and psychological distress by improving an individual's ability to cope with their pain.[193,194] A number of CBT-based interventions have demonstrated effectiveness for improving mental and physical health in individuals with chronic pain[195-197]; however, none to date has examined the efficacy of CBT for chronic pain *specifically among individuals with BD*. In fact, many CBT trials have explicitly excluded individuals with BD and/or other serious mental illnesses.[198-202] Similarly, mindfulness-based interventions—those focused on increasing awareness and acceptance of emotional and physical discomfort—also show promise for individuals with chronic pain,[203-207] though most studies have not focused on or even included individuals with BD. Collaborative care interventions, whereby chronic pain treatment is delivered by a multidisciplinary team often including both behavioral health and internal medicine providers, have made important contributions to the field by often prioritizing patients with comorbid pain and mental health disorders; however, most have focused only on individuals with depression and/or anxiety, excluded those with more serious mental illness,[208-211] or did not report pain-related outcomes among participants with serious mental illness.[212]

Brain stimulation-based treatments such as transcranial magnetic stimulation (TMS), electroconvulsive therapy (ECT), and vagus nerve stimulation (VNS) are receiving increased attention as treatment options for individuals with depressive symptoms and those with pain,[213] although studies have (1) generally focused on major depressive disorder and treatment-resistant depression (and not BD) and (2) examined treatment efficacy for these populations separately. Thus, we do not yet know the impact of these approaches for individuals with comorbid BD and pain.

6.5 Pain and Schizophrenia

6.5.1 Epidemiology

A cross-sectional study of U.S. veterans revealed that pain occurred in 65.6% of patients with depression, 61.3% in those with BD, and 46.9% of those with schizophrenia.[6] Some studies have reported that the prevalence of chronic pain does not significantly differ between those with schizophrenia and the general population in the United States[214] and other countries.[215] However, Owen-Smith and colleagues'[147] analysis of multiple, large, private-sector healthcare systems in the United States revealed that, as compared to patients without a mental health diagnosis, there was a 90% greater risk for a pain diagnosis among those with depression, an 86% greater risk in schizophrenia, and a 71% greater risk in bipolar disorder. Others have observed nearly a fivefold increased risk for chronic pain in BD compared to controls and nearly a fourfold increase among those with schizophrenia.[148]

Experimental pain involves exposing study participants to objective pain stimuli in a controlled laboratory setting. For example, the cold pressure test measures pain tolerance by having participants place their forearm in an ice bath to measure how long they can tolerate the painful stimuli. This type of research has led to some mixed evidence regarding differences in nociception between patients with schizophrenia and healthy controls.[216,217] Similarly, mixed findings have been reported on heat pain tolerance in treated and untreated patients with schizophrenia.[216-219] Two experimental pain studies observed no difference in nociception between patients with and without schizophrenia.[216,217] In addition, heat pain tolerance did not differ within participants tested prior to initiating treatment and 3 days after starting anti psychotics.[216,217] In contrast, two pilot studies investigating the neurophysiology of experimental pain tolerance in patients with schizophrenia reported greater heat pain tolerance among unmedicated patients with schizophrenia compared to healthy controls.[218,219] This was correlated with less activation in pain affective-cognitive processing areas of the brain and hyperactivity in sensory discriminative pain processing regions.[218] Higher heat pain tolerance was observed in unmedicated patients compared to healthy controls, and this did not differ between treated, stable patients with schizophrenia and healthy controls despite non-normal neural pain processing, like that observed in unmedicated patients.[219] Although there have been inconsistent findings regarding experimental pain sensitivity in schizophrenia, the best evidence comes from a large 2015 meta-analyses of 17 studies involving 387 participants.[220] This work revealed patients with schizophrenia, compared to healthy controls, had greater pain tolerance, reduced physiological response to adverse stimuli, and lower pain intensity ratings.[220] These findings were similar in treated and untreated patients.[220]

Because antipsychotics, such as haloperidol, bind to opioid receptors, several studies have compared pain response in patients with versus without antipsychotic treatment.[214] A systematic review of laboratory studies concluded that there is a moderate effect size for diminished pain response, and this is independent of whether patients are receiving antipsychotics.[221] Based on laboratory studies, antipsychotics do not generate sufficient analgesia to change pain perception. Overall, most evidence supports the conclusion that patients with schizophrenia experience greater pain tolerance and report less severe pain when exposed to experimental pain stimuli. Antipsychotic treatment does not significantly change pain perception. Both conclusions are consistent with the few studies of clinical pain in schizophrenia.

However, clinical pain research in schizophrenia raises additional questions. The most common pain locations in schizophrenia are the head, face, abdomen, and lower spinal column.[214] It is alarming that patients with schizophrenia and severe burns, fractures, and myocardial infarction report only minor pain.[214,221,222] Patients with schizophrenia experiencing a myocardial infarction are more likely than persons without schizophrenia to present without pain.[214,222] Consequently, patients may be less likely to report these and other potentially serious conditions to providers,[223] have less help-seeking behaviors,[224] and underutilize appropriate medical care.[225,226]

6.5.2 Impact of Comorbid Chronic Pain and Schizophrenia on Clinical Outcomes

Like patterns observed with other mental health disorders, pain interference is associated with worse global functioning among individuals with schizophrenia.[227] Furthermore, evidence suggests that those with pain have more pronounced symptoms of psychosis, more pronounced depressive symptoms, and larger decrements in health-related quality of life compared to people with psychosis who did not report pain.[228]

6.5.3 Clinical Assessment in Comorbid Chronic Pain and Schizophrenia

Although some evidence suggests a lower prevalence of pain among individuals with schizophrenia (described earlier), this may be because patients are less able to report pain in clinical settings. Impaired executive functioning, attention, and vigilance in individuals with schizophrenia, for example, may contribute to a blunted pain expression.[216] Thus, these patients may experience pain at the same level as healthy controls, as indicated in experimental pain studies, or even at increased levels compared to healthy controls, but they are unable to communicate effectively with their healthcare providers.[229] Given that pain is most commonly assessed through self-report—and requires that the patient (1) understand a provider's request for a pain rating, (2) accurately recall pain events in the given time frame, and (3) accurately interpret the experience of noxious stimuli as a painful event[154]—individuals with serious mental illness (e.g., those with schizophrenia, bipolar disorder, and severe depression) are often unable to adequately describe physical symptoms due to social communication impairments.[230] They may also have lower motivation to report pain to clinicians, perhaps due to concerns about how they will be treated by health-care providers. For example, Kuritzky and colleagues[223] reported that approximately 40% of patients with schizophrenia who had pain-related complaints indicated that they never reported these complaints to avoid being perceived as a burden to clinicians and/or to avoid hospitalization.[214,223] This leads to the possibility that clinical pain is underestimated in schizophrenia because these patients do not seek care for pain.[220] Patients who have experienced inadequate pain management may be reluctant to seek medical care for other health problems as well.[231]

Clinicians may not proactively assess and diagnose pain in patients with serious mental illness as often as with individuals without serious mental illness, and thus pain is likely underrecognized and underdiagnosed in this population. Mental health clinicians may be less likely to assign pain-related diagnoses for individuals with schizophrenia because many have limited training in physical symptom management[232] and are more focused on treating psychiatric than medical concerns[233-235]; primary care clinicians may be less likely to assign pain-related diagnoses because their short consultation times make it difficult to both assess mental symptoms and conduct physical assessments. Additionally, less experienced providers may be uncomfortable with serious mental illness and may avoid intensifying their interaction with a patient by asking probing questions about physical symptoms and performing a physical exam.[232]

The association between experimental and clinical pain and schizophrenia is unique as compared to pain comorbid with other psychiatric disorders. Specifically, there is substantial evidence that persons with schizophrenia have muted pain expression, which could explain the lower pain prevalence observed in this population compared to those with other psychiatric disorders.[6,214] This is consistent with evidence that clinically recognized pain conditions are less common among patients with schizophrenia as compared to patients with depression and bipolar disorder.[6]

6.5.4 Pharmacological Treatment of Comorbid Chronic Pain and Schizophrenia

As discussed earlier, there is a significant overlap in the pharmacological treatment of chronic pain and psychiatric disorders. Second-generation antipsychotics are effective not only for the treatment of patients with schizophrenia who have positive symptoms of psychosis (e.g., delusions, hallucinations, disorganized thoughts and behaviors, perception disturbances, etc.), but also for patients with pain; thus, these medications are particularly useful for patients with comorbid schizophrenia and pain.[236]

It is worth noting that several pharmacological pain treatments are specifically contraindicated for individuals with schizophrenia. For example, though there is evidence that ketamine can be effective at low doses in both acute and chronic pain settings,[237] it can induce delirium and other psychotic symptoms, and thus patients with any history of psychosis are not candidates for ketamine.[238] Also, there have been several case reports of corticosteroid-[239] and opioid-induced[240] psychosis among individuals with no known prior psychiatric histories; thus, caution and additional monitoring may be warranted when using these therapies for patients with schizophrenia and other mental disorders with psychotic symptoms. Finally, as discussed earlier, there has been increasing interest in and use of cannabis for chronic pain; however, a recent overview of systematic reviews reported myriad risks specifically for those at greater risk of or who have diagnoses of schizophrenia and other psychotic disorders. For example, cannabis/cannabinoid use was associated with reduced age at onset of psychosis, increased risk of psychosis onset, diagnosis of schizophrenia/psychotic disorders, transition to psychosis, psychotic symptoms, psychosis relapse/rehospitalization, and non-adherence to antipsychotic medication.[176]

6.5.5 Opioid Therapy in the Context of Comorbid Pain and Schizophrenia

In contrast to findings from studies on individuals with BD, some evidence suggests that individuals with schizophrenia are *not* different from those without psychiatric illness with respect to being prescribed long-term opioid therapy[147]; other studies have reported that patients with psychotic disorders are *less* likely to be prescribed opioids compared to those without any psychiatric illnesses.[241] However, concomitant use of opioids and antipsychotics is not uncommon; about 10–15% of patients are using both medications despite the 2016 FDA "black box" warning about the risks of combining opioids with benzodiazepines and certain (sedating) antipsychotic agents.[242] Indeed, prior studies have reported that, among patients receiving opioids, sedating antipsychotics are associated with a significant increased risk of overdose.[242] This is particularly concerning in the context of evidence that high-risk opioid use (e.g., being in the highest quintile for dose, receiving more than one type of opioid concurrently, receiving concurrent sedative hypnotics, and obtaining early opioid refills) is up to five times more likely among individuals with serious mental illness, such as schizophrenia, compared to the general population.[139]

6.5.6 Non-Pharmacological Management of Comorbid Chronic Pain and Schizophrenia

As described earlier, there is strong evidence for CBT, mindfulness-based interventions, and collaborative care programs for addressing chronic pain. However, many studies documenting the effectiveness of these strategies have excluded individuals with serious mental illness[243] or have not reported outcomes specific to these populations. Indeed, in a review of 98 clinical trials focused on chronic pain, Harris and colleagues[244] report that approximately 16% explicitly excluded individuals with serious mental illness; another review of 75 trials in the 2020 Cochrane review of psychological therapies for pain reported that 60% explicitly excluded individuals with serious mental illness; psychosis or schizophrenia was the most common exclusion.[243] Unfortunately, this significantly impacts our understanding of how those interventions are (or are not) effective for these patients.[244]

There is some promising evidence for the use of virtual reality[245] and deep TMS[246] in reducing pain perception and pain sensation, respectively, among patients with serious mental illness; however, more research is needed to examine the efficacy and potential side effects among those with schizophrenia and across different types of pain conditions.

6.6 Research Gaps and Future Directions for the Study of Comorbid Chronic Pain and Psychiatric Disorders

While several medications and non-pharmacological treatments are used for chronic pain or psychiatric disorders in isolation, treatment trials for patients with chronic pain and psychiatric comorbidity are sparse and represent a significant gap in the literature. This "siloed" individual treatment approach has led to modest treatment effects that need to be addressed with future research. Future studies including novel and larger clinical trials are needed which develop interventions that target comorbidity and test novel care delivery models, such as stepped care, telecare, collaborative care, or integrated (primary care–mental health integration) and interdisciplinary treatment.

To fill the significant literature gap and better guide clinical practice, interventions and care delivery models are needed that address comorbid chronic pain and psychiatric disorders concomitantly rather than as isolated conditions. Comparative effectiveness trials that compare different treatments head to head are lacking and are needed to identify the most effective treatments and which should be prioritized as first and second line. Additionally, implementation studies are necessary to inform how to improve access to evidence-based psychological and behavioral health approaches for patients with both chronic pain and psychiatric disorders.

Since chronic pain and psychiatric comorbidity do not simply co-exist but also interact, it is important to treat these interactions and their combined negative effects.[125,131] Further development and testing of combined interventions that integrate evidence-based psychological, behavioral, and pharmacological treatments to target comorbidity are needed to effectively address both conditions.[247] There are no studies that answer the question if treating chronic pain and psychiatric comorbidity at the same time or sequentially is more effective. Relatedly, it is unknown whether pain and psychiatric outcomes are improved more with separate medical teams or integrated medical teams in the same clinical setting.

Studies are needed to identify implementation strategies that improve access to evidence-based approaches for chronic pain and psychiatric comorbidity and overcome geographical barriers for patients. Other studies are needed to optimize patient engagement, possibly through telehealth, mobile applications, and other technology-facilitated (e.g., virtual reality) interventions. To convince insurers and policymakers to reform unfavorable reimbursement practices for behavioral and psychological interventions, more budget impact analyses and cost effectiveness studies are needed.

6.7 Conclusion

We reviewed the epidemiology of comorbid chronic pain and other psychiatric disorders including anxiety disorders, PTSD, BD, and schizophrenia. Because of the high rates of comorbidity and significant negative impacts on clinical outcomes, we emphasized the importance of clinical assessment of psychiatric conditions in all patients with chronic pain. We highlighted several pharmacological and non-pharmacological treatments that have been used effectively for patients with chronic pain and psychiatric disorders. However, most treatments have been developed for either chronic pain or an individual psychiatric disorder, rather than for their co-occurrence. Future research is needed to develop and test integrated treatments for chronic pain and psychiatric comorbidity.

References

1. Cheatle MD, Gallagher RM. Chronic pain and comorbid mood and substance use disorders: A biopsychosocial treatment approach. *Curr Psychiatry Rep.* 2006;8(5):371–376.
2. Knaster P, Karlsson H, Estlander A-M, Kalso E. Psychiatric disorders as assessed with SCID in chronic pain patients: The anxiety disorders precede the onset of pain. *Gen Hosp Psychiatry.* 2012;34(1):46–52.
3. Otis JD, Keane TM, Kerns RD. An examination of the relationship between chronic pain and post-traumatic stress disorder. *J Rehabil Res Dev.* 2003;40(5):397–405.
4. Bair MJ, Robinson RL, Katon W, Kroenke K. Depression and pain comorbidity: A literature review. *Arch Intern Med.* 2003;163(20):2433–2445.
5. Stubbs B, Eggermont L, Mitchell A, et al. The prevalence of pain in bipolar disorder: A systematic review and large-scale meta-analysis. *Acta Psychiatrica Scandinavica.* 2015;131(2):75–88.
6. Birgenheir DG, Ilgen MA, Bohnert AS, et al. Pain conditions among veterans with schizophrenia or bipolar disorder. *Gen Hosp Psychiatry.* 2013;35(5):480–484.
7. de Heer EW, Gerrits MM, Beekman AT, et al. The association of depression and anxiety with pain: A study from NESDA. *PloS One.* 2014;9(10):e106907.
8. Kessler RC, McGonagle KA, Zhao S, et al. Lifetime and 12-month prevalence of DSM-III-R psychiatric disorders in the United States: Results from the National Comorbidity Survey. *Arch Gen Psychiatry.* 1994;51(1):8–19.
9. Kessler RC, Chiu WT, Demler O, Walters EE. Prevalence, severity, and comorbidity of 12-month DSM-IV disorders in the National Comorbidity Survey Replication. *Arch Gen Psychiatry.* 2005;62(6):617–627.
10. Goldstein-Piekarski A, Williams L, Humphreys K. A trans-diagnostic review of anxiety disorder comorbidity and the impact of multiple exclusion criteria on studying clinical outcomes in anxiety disorders. *Translational Psychiatry.* 2016;6(6):e847–e847.
11. Hirschfeld RM. The comorbidity of major depression and anxiety disorders: Recognition and management in primary care. *Primary Care Companion J Clin Psychiatry.* 2001;3(6):244.
12. Mullins PM, Yong RJ, Bhattacharyya N. Associations between chronic pain, anxiety, and depression among adults in the United States. *Pain Pract.* 2023 Jul;23(6):589–594.
13. Bandelow B. Generalized anxiety disorder and pain. *Pain Psychiatric Disord.* 2015;30:153–165.
14. Atkinson JH, Slater MA, Patterson TL, Grant I, Garfin SR. Prevalence, onset, and risk of psychiatric disorders in men with chronic low back pain: A controlled study. *Pain.* 1991;45(2):111–121.

OTHER PSYCHIATRIC DISORDERS 105

15. Dersh J, Gatchel RJ, Polatin P, Mayer T. Prevalence of psychiatric disorders in patients with chronic work-related musculoskeletal pain disability. *J Occupat Environ Med.* 2002:459–468.
16. Reme SE, Tangen T, Moe T, Eriksen HR. Prevalence of psychiatric disorders in sick listed chronic low back pain patients. *Eur J Pain.* 2011;15(10):1075–1080.
17. Chaturvedi SK. Prevalence of chronic pain in psychiatric patients. *Pain.* 1987;29(2):231–237.
18. Satghare P, Abdin EB, Hombali A, et al. Chronic pain among tertiary care psychiatric outpatients in Singapore: Prevalence and associations with psychiatric disorders. *Pain Res Manag.* 2022 Apr 15:1825132.
19. Rajmohan V, Kumar SK. Psychiatric morbidity, pain perception, and functional status of chronic pain patients in palliative care. *Indian J Palliat Care.* 2013;19(3):146.
20. Workman EA, Hubbard JR, Felker BL. Comorbid psychiatric disorders and predictors of pain management program success in patients with chronic pain. *Primary Care Companion J Clin Psychiatry.* 2002;4(4):137.
21. Bair MJ, Wu J, Damush TM, Sutherland JM, Kroenke K. Association of depression and anxiety alone and in combination with chronic musculoskeletal pain in primary care patients. *Psychosom Med.* 2008;70(8):890.
22. Karp JF, Scott J, Houck P, Reynolds III CF, Kupfer DJ, Frank E. Pain predicts longer time to remission during treatment of recurrent depression. *J Clin Psychiatry.* 2005;66(5):591–597.
23. Bair MJ, Robinson RL, Eckert GJ, Stang PE, Croghan TW, Kroenke K. Impact of pain on depression treatment response in primary care. *Psychosom Med.* 2004;66(1):17–22.
24. Kleykamp BA, Ferguson MC, McNicol E, et al. The Prevalence of Psychiatric and Chronic Pain Comorbidities in Fibromyalgia: An ACTTION systematic review. *Semin Arthritis Rheum.* 2021 Feb;51(1):166–174.
25. Lydiard RB, Falsetti SA. Experience with anxiety and depression treatment studies: Implications for designing irritable bowel syndrome clinical trials. *Am J Med.* 1999;107(5):65–73.
26. Breslau N. Psychiatric comorbidity in migraine. *Cephalalgia.* 1998;18(Suppl 22):56–58; discussion 58.
27. McCracken LM, Iverson GL. Disrupted sleep patterns and daily functioning in patients with chronic pain. *Pain Res Manag.* 2002;7:75–79.
28. Tang NK, Wright KJ, Salkovskis PM. Prevalence and correlates of clinical insomnia co-occurring with chronic back pain. *J Sleep Res.* 2007;16(1):85–95.
29. Büyükyılmaz FE, Şendir M, Acaroğlu R. Evaluation of night-time pain characteristics and quality of sleep in postoperative Turkish orthopedic patients. *Clin Nurs Res.* 2011;20(3):326–342.
30. Tripathi R, Rao R, Dhawan A, Jain R, Sinha S. Opioids and sleep–a review of literature. *Sleep Med.* 2020;67:269–275.
31. Barazzetti L, Garcez A, Sant'Anna PCF, de Bairros FS, Dias-da-Costa JS, Olinto MTA. Does sleep quality modify the relationship between common mental disorders and chronic low back pain in adult women? *Sleep Med.* 2022;96:132–139.
32. Annagür BB, Uguz F, Apiliogullari S, Kara İ, Gunduz S. Psychiatric disorders and association with quality of sleep and quality of life in patients with chronic pain: A SCID-based study. *Pain Med.* 2014;15(5):772–781.
33. Travaglini LE, Cosgrave J, Klingaman EA. Pain and sleep problems predict quality of life for veterans with serious mental illness. *Psychiatric Rehabil J.* 2019;42(3):229.
34. Demyttenaere K, Bruffaerts R, Lee S, et al. Mental disorders among persons with chronic back or neck pain: Results from the World Mental Health Surveys. *Pain.* 2007;129(3):332–342.

35. Goral A, Lipsitz JD, Gross R. The relationship of chronic pain with and without comorbid psychiatric disorder to sleep disturbance and health care utilization: Results from the Israel National Health Survey. *J Psychosom Res.* 2010;69(5):449–457.
36. McWilliams LA, Cox BJ, Enns MW. Mood and anxiety disorders associated with chronic pain: An examination in a nationally representative sample. *Pain.* 2003;106(1–2):127–133.
37. Von Korff M, Crane P, Lane M, et al. Chronic spinal pain and physical–mental comorbidity in the United States: Results from the national comorbidity survey replication. *Pain.* 2005;113(3):331–339.
38. Husak AJ, Bair MJ. Chronic pain and sleep disturbances: A pragmatic review of their relationships, comorbidities, and treatments. *Pain Med.* 2020;21(6):1142–1152.
39. Asmundson GJ, Katz J. Understanding the co-occurrence of anxiety disorders and chronic pain: State-of-the-art. *Depression Anxiety.* 2009;26(10):888–901.
40. Fishbain DA, Goldberg M, Labbé E, Steele R, Rosomoff H. Compensation and non-compensation chronic pain patients compared for DSM-III operational diagnoses. *Pain.* 1988;32(2):197–206.
41. Gerhardt A, Hartmann M, Schuller-Roma B, et al. The prevalence and type of Axis-I and Axis-II mental disorders in subjects with non-specific chronic back pain: Results from a population-based study. *Pain Med.* 2011;12(8):1231–1240.
42. Remes O, Brayne C, Van Der Linde R, Lafortune L. A systematic review of reviews on the prevalence of anxiety disorders in adult populations. *Brain Behav.* 2016;6(7):e00497.
43. Swartz KL, Pratt LA, Armenian HK, Lee LC, Eaton WW. Mental disorders and the incidence of migraine headaches in a community sample: Results from the Baltimore Epidemiologic Catchment area follow-up study. *Arch Gen Psychiatry.* 2000;57(10):945–950.
44. Raphael KG, Janal MN, Nayak S, Schwartz JE, Gallagher RM. Psychiatric comorbidities in a community sample of women with fibromyalgia. *Pain.* 2006;124(1–2):117–125.
45. Kroenke K, Outcalt S, Krebs E, et al. Association between anxiety, health-related quality of life and functional impairment in primary care patients with chronic pain. *Gen Hosp Psychiatry.* 2013;35(4):359–365.
46. Romão APMS, Gorayeb R, Romão GS, et al. High levels of anxiety and depression have a negative effect on quality of life of women with chronic pelvic pain. *Int J Clin Pract.* 2009;63(5):707–711.
47. Kuch K, Cox BJ, Woszczyna CB, Swinson RP, Shulman I. Chronic pain in panic disorder. *J Behav Ther Exp Psychiatry.* 1991;22(4):255–259.
48. Kinney RK, Gatchel RJ, Polatin PB, Fogarty WT, Mayer TG. Prevalence of psychopathology in acute and chronic low back pain patients. *J Occupat Rehabil.* 1993;3:95–103.
49. McWilliams LA, Goodwin RD, Cox BJ. Depression and anxiety associated with three pain conditions: Results from a nationally representative sample. *Pain.* 2004;111(1–2):77–83.
50. Zamani M, Alizadeh-Tabari S, Zamani V. Systematic review with meta-analysis: The prevalence of anxiety and depression in patients with irritable bowel syndrome. *Alimentary Pharmacol Therapeutics.* 2019;50(2):132–143.
51. Kroenke K, Spitzer RL, Williams J, et al. Physical symptoms in primary care. Predictors of psychiatric disorders and functional impairment. *Arch Fam Med.* 1994;3(9):774–779.
52. Means-Christensen AJ, Roy-Byrne PP, Sherbourne CD, Craske MG, Stein MB. Relationships among pain, anxiety, and depression in primary care. *Depression Anxiety.* 2008;25(7):593–600.
53. Rhudy JL, Meagher MW. Fear and anxiety: Divergent effects on human pain thresholds. *Pain.* 2000;84(1):65–75.
54. Beynon AM, Hebert JJ, Hodgetts CJ, Boulos LM, Walker BF. Chronic physical illnesses, mental health disorders, and psychological features as potential risk factors for back pain from childhood to young adulthood: A systematic review with meta-analysis. *Eur Spine J.* 2020;29:480–496.

OTHER PSYCHIATRIC DISORDERS 107

55. Ferguson RJ, Ahles TA. Private body consciousness, anxiety and pain symptom reports of chronic pain patients. *Behav Res Ther.* 1998;36(5):527–535.
56. Woo AK. Depression and anxiety in pain. *Rev Pain.* 2010;4(1):8–12.
57. Blozik E, Laptinskaya D, Herrmann-Lingen C, et al. Depression and anxiety as major determinants of neck pain: A cross-sectional study in general practice. *BMC Musculoskel Disord.* 2009;10(1):1–8.
58. Varni JW, Rapoff MA, Waldron SA, Gragg RA, Bernstein BH, Lindsley CB. Chronic pain and emotional distress in children and adolescents. *J Dev Behav Pediatr.* 1996;17(3):154–161.
59. Pangarkar SS, Kang DG, Sandbrink F, et al. VA/DoD clinical practice guideline: Diagnosis and treatment of low back pain. *J Gen Intern Med.* 2019;34:2620–2629.
60. Sandbrink F, Murphy JL, Johansson M, et al. The use of opioids in the management of chronic pain: Synopsis of the 2022 Updated US Department of Veterans Affairs and US Department of Defense clinical practice guideline. *Ann Intern Med.* 2023;176(3):388–397.
61. Sharma A, Kudesia P, Shi Q, Gandhi R. Anxiety and depression in patients with osteoarthritis: Impact and management challenges. *Open Access Rheumatol Res Rev.* 2016:103–113.
62. El-Gabalawy R, Mackenzie CS, Shooshtari S, Sareen J. Comorbid physical health conditions and anxiety disorders: A population-based exploration of prevalence and health outcomes among older adults. *General Hosp Psychiatry.* 2011;33(6):556–564.
63. Teh CF, Morone NE, Karp JF, et al. Pain interference impacts response to treatment for anxiety disorders. *Depression Anxiety.* 2009;26(3):222–228.
64. Engel GL. The need for a new medical model: A challenge for biomedicine. *Science.* 1977;196(4286):129–136.
65. Krebs EE, Lorenz KA, Bair MJ, et al. Development and initial validation of the PEG, a three-item scale assessing pain intensity and interference. *J Gen Intern Med.* 2009;24:733–738.
66. Sherbourne CD, Asch SM, Shugarman LR, et al. Early identification of co-occurring pain, depression and anxiety. *J Gen Intern Med* 2009;24:620–625.
67. Vermani M, Marcus M, Katzman MA. Rates of detection of mood and anxiety disorders in primary care: A descriptive, cross-sectional study. *Primary Care Companion CNS Disord.* 2011;13(2):27211.
68. Jordan KD, Okifuji A. Anxiety disorders: Differential diagnosis and their relationship to chronic pain. *J Pain Palliat Care Pharmacother.* 2011;25(3):231–245.
69. Kroenke K, Spitzer RL, Williams JB, Monahan PO, Löwe B. Anxiety disorders in primary care: Prevalence, impairment, comorbidity, and detection. *Ann Intern Med.* 2007;146(5):317–325.
70. Spitzer RL, Kroenke K, Williams JB, Löwe B. A brief measure for assessing generalized anxiety disorder: The GAD-7. *Arch Intern Med.* 2006;166(10):1092–1097.
71. Zigmond AS, Snaith RP. The hospital anxiety and depression scale. *Acta Psychiatrica Scandinavica.* 1983;67(6):361–370.
72. McCracken LM, Zayfert C, Gross RT. The Pain Anxiety Symptoms Scale: Development and validation of a scale to measure fear of pain. *Pain.* 1992;50(1):67–73.
73. Management ASoATFoCP. Practice guidelines for chronic pain management: An updated report by the American Society of Anesthesiologists Task Force on Chronic Pain Management and the American Society of Regional Anesthesia and Pain Medicine. *Anesthesiology.* 2010;112(4):810–833.
74. Baldwin DS, Anderson IM, Nutt DJ, et al. Evidence-based pharmacological treatment of anxiety disorders, post-traumatic stress disorder and obsessive-compulsive disorder: A revision of the 2005 guidelines from the British Association for Psychopharmacology. *J Psychopharmacol.* 2014;28(5):403–439.
75. Gautam S, Jain A, Gautam M, Vahia VN, Gautam A. Clinical practice guidelines for the management of generalised anxiety disorder (GAD) and panic disorder (PD). *Indian J Psychiatry.* 2017;59(Suppl 1):S67.

76. Cassano GB, Rossi NB, Pini S. Psychopharmacology of anxiety disorders. *Dialogues Clin Neurosci.* 2002 Sep;4(3):271–285.
77. Melaragno AJ. Pharmacotherapy for anxiety disorders: From first-line options to treatment resistance. *Focus.* 2021;19(2):145–160.
78. Bandelow B, Michaelis S, Wedekind D. Treatment of anxiety disorders. *Dialogues Clin Neurosci.* 2017 Jun;19(2):93–107.
79. Patetsos E, Horjales-Araujo E. Treating chronic pain with SSRIs: What do we know? *Pain Research and Manag.* 2016;2016:2020915.
80. O'Malley PG, Jackson JL, Santoro J, Tomkins G, Balden E, Kroenke K. Antidepressant therapy for unexplained symptoms and symptom syndromes. *J Fam Pract.* 1999 Dec;48(12):980–990.
81. Clauw DJ, Crofford LJ. Chronic widespread pain and fibromyalgia: What we know, and what we need to know. *Best Pract Res Clin Rheumatol.* 2003;17(4):685–701.
82. Lee Y-C, Chen P-P. A review of SSRIs and SNRIs in neuropathic pain. *Exp Opin Pharmacother.* 2010;11(17):2813–2825.
83. Max MB, Lynch SA, Muir J, Shoaf SE, Smoller B, Dubner R. Effects of desipramine, amitriptyline, and fluoxetine on pain in diabetic neuropathy. *N Engl J Med.* 1992;326(19):1250–1256.
84. Jackson JL, Mancuso JM, Nickoloff S, Bernstein R, Kay C. Tricyclic and tetracyclic antidepressants for the prevention of frequent episodic or chronic tension-type headache in adults: A systematic review and meta-analysis. *J Gen Intern Med.* 2017;32:1351–1358.
85. Ferreira GE, Abdel-Shaheed C, Underwood M, et al. Efficacy, safety, and tolerability of antidepressants for pain in adults: Overview of systematic reviews. *BMJ.* 2023;380.
86. Raskin J, Pritchett YL, Wang F, et al. A double-blind, randomized multicenter trial comparing duloxetine with placebo in the management of diabetic peripheral neuropathic pain. *Pain Med.* 2005;6(5):346–356.
87. Goldstein DJ, Lu Y, Detke MJ, Lee TC, Iyengar S. Duloxetine vs. placebo in patients with painful diabetic neuropathy. *Pain.* 2005;116(1–2):109–118.
88. Wernicke J, Pritchett Y, D'souza D, et al. A randomized controlled trial of duloxetine in diabetic peripheral neuropathic pain. *Neurology.* 2006;67(8):1411–1420.
89. Lunn MP, Hughes RA, Wiffen PJ. Duloxetine for treating painful neuropathy, chronic pain or fibromyalgia. *Cochrane Database Syst Rev.* 2014(1).
90. Gallagher HC, Gallagher RM, Butler M, Buggy DJ, Henman MC. Venlafaxine for neuropathic pain in adults. *Cochrane Database Syst Rev.* 2015(8).
91. Hong JS, Atkinson LZ, Al-Juffali N, et al. Gabapentin and pregabalin in bipolar disorder, anxiety states, and insomnia: Systematic review, meta-analysis, and rationale. *Molec Psychiatry.* 2022;27(3):1339–1349.
92. Senderovich H, Jeyapragasan G. Is there a role for combined use of gabapentin and pregabalin in pain control? Too good to be true? *Curr Med Res Opin.* 2018;34(4):677–682.
93. Harirforoosh S, Asghar W, Jamali F. Adverse effects of nonsteroidal antiinflammatory drugs: An update of gastrointestinal, cardiovascular and renal complications. *J Pharm Pharmaceut Sci.* 2013;16(5):821–847.
94. Wongrakpanich S, Wongrakpanich A, Melhado K, Rangaswami J. A comprehensive review of non-steroidal anti-inflammatory drug use in the elderly. *Aging Dis.* 2018;9(1):143.
95. De Jong JC, Van Den Berg PB, Tobi H, De Jong LT. Combined use of SSRIs and NSAIDs increases the risk of gastrointestinal adverse effects. *Br J Clin Pharmacol.* 2003;55(6):591–595.
96. Ragheb M. The clinical significance of lithium-nonsteroidal anti-inflammatory drug interactions. *J Clin Psychopharmacol.* 1990;10(5):350–354.
97. Van Rijswijk S, van Beek M, Schoof G, Schene A, Steegers M, Schellekens A. Iatrogenic opioid use disorder, chronic pain and psychiatric comorbidity: A systematic review. *Gen Hosp Psychiatry.* 2019;59:37–50.

OTHER PSYCHIATRIC DISORDERS   109

98. Reisfield GM, Webster LR. Benzodiazepines in long-term opioid therapy. *Pain Med.* 2013;14(10):1441–1446.

99. Parthipan A, Banerjee I, Humphreys K, et al. Predicting inadequate postoperative pain management in depressed patients: A machine learning approach. *PLoS One.* 2019;14(2):e0210575.

100. Geneen LJ, Martin DJ, Adams N, et al. Effects of education to facilitate knowledge about chronic pain for adults: A systematic review with meta-analysis. *Systematic Rev.* 2015;4(1):1–21.

101. Morley S. Efficacy and effectiveness of cognitive behaviour therapy for chronic pain: Progress and some challenges. *Pain.* 2011;152(3):S99–S106.

102. Curtiss JE, Levine DS, Ander I, Baker AW. Cognitive-behavioral treatments for anxiety and stress-related disorders. *Focus.* 2021;19(2):184–189.

103. Proctor SL, Estroff TW, Empting LD, Shearer-Williams S, Hoffmann NG. Prevalence of substance use and psychiatric disorders in a highly select chronic pain population. *J Addiction Med.* 2013;7(1):17–24.

104. Akhtar E, Ballew AT, Orr WN, Mayorga A, Khan TW. The prevalence of post-traumatic stress disorder symptoms in chronic pain patients in a tertiary care setting: A cross-sectional study. *Psychosomatics.* 2019;60(3):255–262.

105. Hickling EJ, Blanchard EB, Silverman DJ, Schwarz SR. Motor vehicle accidents, headaches and post-traumatic stress disorder: Assessment findings in a consecutive series. *Headache.* 1992;32(3):147–151.

106. Asmundson GJ, Norton GR, Allerdings MD, Norton PJ, Larsen DK. Posttraumatic stress disorder and work-related injury. *J Anxiety Disord.* 1998;12(1):57–69.

107. Häuser W, Galek A, Erbslöh-Möller B, et al. Posttraumatic stress disorder in fibromyalgia syndrome: Prevalence, temporal relationship between posttraumatic stress and fibromyalgia symptoms, and impact on clinical outcome. *Pain.* 2013;154(8):1216–1223.

108. McFarlane AC, Atchison M, Rafalowicz E, Papay P. Physical symptoms in post-traumatic stress disorder. *J Psychosom Res.* 1994;38(7):715–726.

109. Lew HL, Cifu DX, Hinds SR. National prevalence of traumatic brain injury, posttraumatic stress disorder, and pain diagnoses in OIF/OEF/OND Veterans from 2009 to 2011. *J Rehabil Res Dev.* 2013;50(9):xi.

110. Asmundson GJ, Coons MJ, Taylor S, Katz J. PTSD and the experience of pain: Research and clinical implications of shared vulnerability and mutual maintenance models. *Can J Psychiatry.* 2002;47(10):930–937.

111. Beckham JC, Crawford AL, Feldman ME, et al. Chronic posttraumatic stress disorder and chronic pain in Vietnam combat veterans. *J Psychosom Res* 1997;43(4):379–389.

112. White P, Faustman W. Coexisting physical conditions among inpatients with post-traumatic stress disorder. *Military Med.* 1989;154(2):66–71.

113. McWilliams LA, Higgins KS. Associations between pain conditions and borderline personality disorder symptoms: Findings from the National Comorbidity Survey Replication. *Clin J Pain.* 2013;29(6):527–532.

114. Noel M, Vinall J, Tomfohr-Madsen L, Holley AL, Wilson AC, Palermo TM. Sleep mediates the association between PTSD symptoms and chronic pain in youth. *J Pain.* 2018;19(1):67–75.

115. Ohayon MM, Shapiro CM. Posttraumatic stress disorder in the general population. *Comprehen Psychiatry.* 2000;41(6):469–478.

116. Lang KP, Veazey-Morris K, Andrasik F. Exploring the role of insomnia in the relation between PTSD and pain in veterans with polytrauma injuries. *J Head Trauma Rehabil.* 2014;29(1):44–53.

117. Benedict TM, Keenan PG, Nitz AJ, Moeller-Bertram T. Post-traumatic stress disorder symptoms contribute to worse pain and health outcomes in veterans with PTSD compared to those without: A systematic review with meta-analysis. *Military Med.* 2020;185(9-10):e1481–e1491.

118. Edlund MJ, Steffick D, Hudson T, Harris KM, Sullivan M. Risk factors for clinically recognized opioid abuse and dependence among veterans using opioids for chronic non-cancer pain. *Pain.* 2007;129(3):355–362.
119. Morasco BJ, O'Hearn D, Turk DC, Dobscha SK. Associations between prescription opioid use and sleep impairment among veterans with chronic pain. *Pain Med.* 2014;15(11):1902–1910.
120. Sherman JJ, Turk DC, Okifuji A. Prevalence and impact of posttraumatic stress disorder-like symptoms on patients with fibromyalgia syndrome. *Clinical J Pain.* 2000;16(2):127–134.
121. Villano CL, Rosenblum A, Magura S, Fong C, Cleland C, Betzler TF. Prevalence and correlates of posttraumatic stress disorder and chronic severe pain in psychiatric outpatients. *J Rehabil Res Dev.* 2007;44(2):167–178.
122. Geisser ME, Roth RS, Bachman JE, Eckert TA. The relationship between symptoms of post-traumatic stress disorder and pain, affective disturbance and disability among patients with accident and non-accident related pain. *PAIN®.* 1996;66(2–3):207–214.
123. Ang DC, Wu J, Sargent C, Bair MJ. Pain experience of Iraq and Afghanistan Veterans with comorbid chronic pain and posttraumatic stress. *J Rehabil Res Dev.* 2014;51(4):559.
124. Beck JG, Gudmundsdottir B, Shipherd JC. PTSD and emotional distress symptoms measured after a motor vehicle accident: Relationships with pain coping profiles. *J Psychopathol Behav Assess.* 2003;25:219–227.
125. Clapp JD, Beck JG, Palyo SA, Grant DM. An examination of the synergy of pain and PTSD on quality of life: Additive or multiplicative effects? *Pain.* 2008;138(2):301–309.
126. Sharp TJ, Harvey AG. Chronic pain and posttraumatic stress disorder: Mutual maintenance? *Clin Psychol Rev.* 2001;21(6):857–877.
127. Alschuler KN, Otis JD. Coping strategies and beliefs about pain in veterans with co-morbid chronic pain and significant levels of posttraumatic stress disorder symptoms. *Eur J Pain.* 2012;16(2):312–319.
128. Palyo SA, Beck GJ. Post-traumatic stress disorder symptoms, pain, and perceived life control: Associations with psychosocial and physical functioning. *Pain.* 2005;117(1):121–127.
129. Blakey SM, Wagner HR, Naylor J, et al. Chronic pain, TBI, and PTSD in military veterans: A link to suicidal ideation and violent impulses? *J Pain.* 2018;19(7):797–806.
130. Beck JG, Clapp JD. A different kind of comorbidity: Understanding posttraumatic stress disorder and chronic pain. *Psychol Trauma.* 2011;3(2):101.
131. Helmer DA, Chandler HK, Quigley KS, Blatt M, Teichman R, Lange G. Chronic widespread pain, mental health, and physical role function in OEF/OIF veterans. *Pain Med.* 2009;10(7):1174–1182.
132. Weathers FW, Bovin MJ, Lee DJ, et al. The Clinician-Administered PTSD Scale for DSM-5 (CAPS-5): Development and initial psychometric evaluation in military veterans. *Psychol Assess.* 2018;30(3):383.
133. Blevins CA, Weathers FW, Davis MT, Witte TK, Domino JL. The posttraumatic stress disorder checklist for DSM-5 (PCL-5): Development and initial psychometric evaluation. *J Trauma Stress.* 2015;28(6):489–498.
134. Marx BP, Lee DJ, Norman SB, et al. Reliable and clinically significant change in the clinician-administered PTSD Scale for DSM-5 and PTSD Checklist for DSM-5 among male veterans. *Psychol Assess.* 2022;34(2):197.
135. Jeffreys M, Bruce Capehart MD M, Friedman MJ. Pharmacotherapy for posttraumatic stress disorder: Review with clinical applications. *J Rehabil Res Dev.* 2012;49(5):703.
136. Zhang Z-X, Liu R-B, Zhang J, et al. Clinical outcomes of recommended active pharmacotherapy agents from NICE guideline for post-traumatic stress disorder: Network meta-analysis. *Prog Neuro-Psychopharmacol Biol Psychiatry.* 2023;125:110754.
137. Nappi CM, Drummond SP, Hall JM. Treating nightmares and insomnia in posttraumatic stress disorder: A review of current evidence. *Neuropharmacology.* 2012;62(2):576–585.

OTHER PSYCHIATRIC DISORDERS 111

138. Committee SoP, Aurora RN, Zak RS, et al. Best practice guide for the treatment of nightmare disorder in adults. *J Clin Sleep Med.* 2010;6(4):389–401.

139. Seal KH, Shi Y, Cohen G, et al. Association of mental health disorders with prescription opioids and high-risk opioid use in US veterans of Iraq and Afghanistan. *JAMA.* 2012;307(9):940–947.

140. Seal KH, Maguen S, Bertenthal D, et al. Observational evidence for buprenorphine's impact on posttraumatic stress symptoms in veterans with chronic pain and opioid use disorder. *J Clin Psychiatry.* 2016;77(9):2154.

141. Forman-Hoffman V, Middleton JC, Feltner C, et al. Psychological and pharmacological treatments for adults with posttraumatic stress disorder: A systematic review update [internet]. Agency for Healthcare Research and Quality (US); 2018 May. Report No.: 18-EHC011-EFReport No.: 2018-SR-01. PMID: 30204376.

142. Susskind O, Friedman MJ. The VA/DOD clinical practice guideline for management of post-traumatic stress (update 2010): Development and methodology. *J Rehabil Res Dev.* 2012;49(5):17.

143. Sharp TJ. The prevalence of post-traumatic stress disorder in chronic pain patients. *Curr Pain Headache Rep.* 2004;8:111–115.

144. Shipherd JC, Beck JG, Hamblen JL, Lackner JM, Freeman JB. A preliminary examination of treatment for posttraumatic stress disorder in chronic pain patients: A case study. *J Trauma Stress.* 2003;16:451–457.

145. Shipherd JC, Keyes M, Jovanovic T, et al. Veterans seeking treatment for posttraumatic stress disorder: What about comorbid chronic pain? *J Rehabil Res Dev.* 2007;44(2):153–166.

146. Nicholl BI, Mackay D, Cullen B, et al. Chronic multisite pain in major depression and bipolar disorder: Cross-sectional study of 149,611 participants in UK Biobank. *BMC Psychiatry.* 2014;14:1–11.

147. Owen-Smith A, Stewart C, Sesay MM, et al. Chronic pain diagnoses and opioid dispensings among insured individuals with serious mental illness. *BMC Psychiatry.* 2020;20:1–10.

148. Bahorik AL, Satre DD, Kline-Simon AH, Weisner CM, Campbell CI. Serious mental illness and medical comorbidities: Findings from an integrated health care system. *J Psychosom Res.* 2017;100:35–45.

149. McIntyre RS, Konarski JZ, Wilkins K, Bouffard B, Soczynska JK, Kennedy SH. The prevalence and impact of migraine headache in bipolar disorder: Results from the Canadian Community Health Survey: CME. *Headache.* 2006;46(6):973–982.

150. Oedegaard KJ, Fasmer OB. Is migraine in unipolar depressed patients a bipolar spectrum trait? *J Affect Disord.* 2005;84(2-3):233–242.

151. Failde I, Dueñas M, Agüera-Ortíz L, Cervilla JA, Gonzalez-Pinto A, Mico JA. Factors associated with chronic pain in patients with bipolar depression: A cross-sectional study. *BMC Psychiatry.* 2013;13:1–7.

152. Hester J, Tang NK. Insomnia co-occurring with chronic pain: Clinical features, interaction, assessments and possible interventions. *Rev Pain.* 2008;2(1):2–7.

153. Jackson A, Cavanagh J, Scott J. A systematic review of manic and depressive prodromes. *J Affect Disord.* 2003;74(3):209–217.

154. De Hert M, Correll CU, Bobes J, et al. Physical illness in patients with severe mental disorders. I. Prevalence, impact of medications and disparities in health care. *World Psychiatry.* 2011;10(1):52.

155. Elman I, Zubieta J-K, Borsook D. The missing p in psychiatric training: Why it is important to teach pain to psychiatrists. *Arch Gen Psychiatry.* 2011;68(1):12–20.

156. Miller CJ, Abraham KM, Bajor LA, et al. Quality of life among patients with bipolar disorder in primary care versus community mental health settings. *J Affect Disord.* 2013;146(1):100–105.

157. Hirschfeld RM, Calabrese JR, Weissman MM, et al. Screening for bipolar disorder in the community. *J Clin Psychiatry.* 2003;64(1):53–59.

158. Ratcliffe GE, Enns MW, Belik S-L, Sareen J. Chronic pain conditions and suicidal ideation and suicide attempts: An epidemiologic perspective. *Clin J Pain.* 2008;24(3):204–210.

159. Risch N, Dubois J, M'bailara K, et al. Self-reported pain and emotional reactivity in bipolar disorder: A prospective face-bd study. *J Clin Med.* 2022;11(3):893.

160. Travaglini LE, Kuykendall L, Bennett ME, Abel EA, Lucksted A. Relationships between chronic pain and mood symptoms among veterans with bipolar disorder. *J Affect Disord.* 2020;277:765–771.

161. Boggero IA, Cole JD. Mania reduces perceived pain intensity in patients with chronic pain: Preliminary evidence from retrospective archival data. *J Pain Res.* 2016:147–152.

162. Minichino A, Delle Chiaie R, Cruccu G, et al. Pain-processing abnormalities in bipolar I disorder, bipolar II disorder, and schizophrenia: A novel trait marker for psychosis proneness and functional outcome? *Bipolar Disord.* 2016;18(7):591–601.

163. Sidhu HS, Sadhotra A. Current status of the new antiepileptic drugs in chronic pain. *Front Pharmacol.* 2016;7:276.

164. Arnold LM. Management of psychiatric comorbidity in fibromyalgia. *Curr Psychiatry Rep.* 2006;8:241–245.

165. Pacchiarotti I, Bond DJ, Baldessarini RJ, et al. The International Society for Bipolar Disorders (ISBD) task force report on antidepressant use in bipolar disorders. *Am J Psychiatry.* 2013;170(11):1249–1262.

166. Saarto T, Wiffen PJ. Antidepressants for neuropathic pain: A Cochrane review. *J Neurol Neurosurg Psychiatry.* 2010;81(12):1372–1373.

167. Bjordal JM, Klovning A, Ljunggren AE, Slørdal L. Short-term efficacy of pharmacotherapeutic interventions in osteoarthritic knee pain: A meta-analysis of randomised placebo-controlled trials. *Eur J Pain.* 2007;11(2):125–138.

168. Finnerup NB, Sindrup SH, Jensen TS. The evidence for pharmacological treatment of neuropathic pain. *Pain.* 2010;150(3):573–581.

169. Machado GC, Maher CG, Ferreira PH, et al. Efficacy and safety of paracetamol for spinal pain and osteoarthritis: Systematic review and meta-analysis of randomised placebo controlled trials. *BMJ.* 2015 Mar 31;350:h1225.

170. Machado L, Kamper S, Herbert R, Maher C, McAuley J. Analgesic effects of treatments for non-specific low back pain: A meta-analysis of placebo-controlled randomized trials. *Rheumatology.* 2009;48(5):520–527.

171. Broekmans S, Dobbels F, Milisen K, Morlion B, Vanderschueren S. Pharmacologic pain treatment in a multidisciplinary pain center: Do patients adhere to the prescription of the physician? *Clin J Pain.* 2010;26(2):81–86.

172. Lynch ME, Cesar-Rittenberg P, Hohmann AG. A double-blind, placebo-controlled, crossover pilot trial with extension using an oral mucosal cannabinoid extract for treatment of chemotherapy-induced neuropathic pain. *J Pain Sympt Manag.* 2014;47(1):166–173.

173. Attal N, Cruccu G, Haanpää M, et al. EFNS guidelines on pharmacological treatment of neuropathic pain. *Eur J Neurol.* 2006;13(11):1153–1169.

174. Moulin D, Boulanger A, Clark A, et al. Pharmacological management of chronic neuropathic pain: Revised consensus statement from the Canadian Pain Society. *Pain Res Manag.* 2014;19:328–335.

175. Cougle JR, Hakes JK, Macatee RJ, Chavarria J, Zvolensky MJ. Quality of life and risk of psychiatric disorders among regular users of alcohol, nicotine, and cannabis: An analysis of the National Epidemiological Survey on Alcohol and Related Conditions (NESARC). *J Psychiatric Res.* 2015;66:135–141.

176. Mohiuddin M, Blyth FM, Degenhardt L, et al. General risks of harm with cannabinoids, cannabis, and cannabis-based medicine possibly relevant to patients receiving these for pain management: An overview of systematic reviews. *Pain.* 2021;162:S80–S96.

177. Braden JB, Sullivan MD, Ray GT, et al. Trends in long-term opioid therapy for noncancer pain among persons with a history of depression. *Gen Hosp Psychiatry.* 2009;31(6):564–570.
178. Davis MA, Lin LA, Liu H, Sites BD. Prescription opioid use among adults with mental health disorders in the United States. *J Am Board Fam Med.* 2017;30(4):407–417.
179. Mathew N, Rosenheck RA. Prescription opioid use among seriously mentally ill veterans nationally in the veterans health administration. *Commun Mental Health J.* 2016;52:165–173.
180. Merrill JO, Von Korff M, Banta-Green CJ, et al. Prescribed opioid difficulties, depression and opioid dose among chronic opioid therapy patients. *Gen Hosp Psychiatry.* 2012;34(6):581–587.
181. Spivak S, Cullen B, Eaton W, et al. Prescription opioid use among individuals with serious mental illness. *Psychiatry Res.* 2018;267:85–87.
182. Sullivan MD, Edlund MJ, Zhang L, Unützer J, Wells KB. Association between mental health disorders, problem drug use, and regular prescription opioid use. *Arch Intern Med.* 2006;166(19):2087–2093.
183. Wasan AD, Davar G, Jamison R. The association between negative affect and opioid analgesia in patients with discogenic low back pain. *Pain.* 2005;117(3):450–461.
184. Goesling J, Henry MJ, Moser SE, et al. Symptoms of depression are associated with opioid use regardless of pain severity and physical functioning among treatment-seeking patients with chronic pain. *J Pain.* 2015;16(9):844–851.
185. Schaffer CB, Nordahl TE, Schaffer LC, Howe J. Mood-elevating effects of opioid analgesics in patients with bipolar disorder. *J Neuropsychiatry Clin Neurosci.* 2007;19(4):449–452.
186. Martins SS, Keyes KM, Storr CL, Zhu H, Chilcoat HD. Pathways between nonmedical opioid use/dependence and psychiatric disorders: Results from the National Epidemiologic Survey on Alcohol and Related Conditions. *Drug Alcohol Depend.* 2009;103(1–2):16–24.
187. Chen K-J, Lu M-L, Shen WW. Tramadol-related psychosis in a patient with bipolar I disorder. *Acta Neuropsychiatrica.* 2015;27(2):126–128.
188. Leung J, Santo Jr T, Colledge-Frisby S, et al. Mood and anxiety symptoms in persons taking prescription opioids: A systematic review with meta-analyses of longitudinal studies. *Pain Med.* 2022;23(8):1442–1456.
189. Schepis TS, Hakes JK. Dose-related effects for the precipitation of psychopathology by opioid or tranquilizer/sedative nonmedical prescription use: Results from the National Epidemiologic Survey on Alcohol and Related Conditions. *J Addiction Med.* 2013;7(1):39–44.
190. Wasan AD, Butler SF, Budman SH, Benoit C, Fernandez K, Jamison RN. Psychiatric history and psychologic adjustment as risk factors for aberrant drug-related behavior among patients with chronic pain. *Clin J Pain.* 2007;23(4):307–315.
191. Carroll CP, Haythornthwaite J. Maladaptive opioid use behaviors and psychiatric illness: What should we do with what we know? *Curr Pain Headache Rep.* 2011;15:91–93.
192. Liebschutz JM, Saitz R, Weiss RD, et al. Clinical factors associated with prescription drug use disorder in urban primary care patients with chronic pain. *J Pain.* 2010;11(11):1047–1055.
193. Ehde DM, Dillworth TM, Turner JA. Cognitive-behavioral therapy for individuals with chronic pain: Efficacy, innovations, and directions for research. *Am Psychol.* 2014;69(2):153.
194. Kerns RD, Sellinger J, Goodin BR. Psychological treatment of chronic pain. *Ann Rev Clin Psychol.* 2011;7:411–434.
195. Hajihasani A, Rouhani M, Salavati M, Hedayati R, Kahlaee AH. The influence of cognitive behavioral therapy on pain, quality of life, and depression in patients receiving physical therapy for chronic low back pain: A systematic review. *PM R.* 2019;11(2):167–176.

196. Knoerl R, Lavoie Smith EM, Weisberg J. Chronic pain and cognitive behavioral therapy: An integrative review. *West J Nurs Res*. 2016;38(5):596–628.
197. Mariano TY, Urman RD, Hutchison CA, Jamison RN, Edwards RR. Cognitive behavioral therapy (CBT) for subacute low back pain: A systematic review. *Curr Pain Headache Rep*. 2018;22:1–7.
198. Darnall BD, Roy A, Chen AL, et al. Comparison of a single-session pain management skills intervention with a single-session health education intervention and 8 sessions of cognitive behavioral therapy in adults with chronic low back pain: A randomized clinical trial. *JAMA Netw Open*. 2021;4(8):e2113401–e2113401.
199. Vibe Fersum K, O'Sullivan P, Skouen J, Smith A, Kvåle A. Efficacy of classification-based cognitive functional therapy in patients with non-specific chronic low back pain: A randomized controlled trial. *Eur J Pain*. 2013;17(6):916–928.
200. Flor H, Birbaumer N. Comparison of the efficacy of electromyographic biofeedback, cognitive-behavioral therapy, and conservative medical interventions in the treatment of chronic musculoskeletal pain. *J Consult Clin Psychol*. 1993;61(4):653.
201. Dysvik E, Kvaløy JT, Natvig GK. The effectiveness of an improved multidisciplinary pain management programme: A 6-and 12-month follow-up study. *J Advance Nurs*. 2012;68(5):1061–1072.
202. Kristjánsdóttir ÓB, Fors EA, Eide E, et al. A smartphone-based intervention with diaries and therapist-feedback to reduce catastrophizing and increase functioning in women with chronic widespread pain: Randomized controlled trial. *J Med Internet Res*. 2013;15(1):e5.
203. Ball EF, Sharizan ENSM, Franklin G, Rogozińska E. Does mindfulness meditation improve chronic pain? A systematic review. *Curr Opin Obstetr Gynecol*.2017;29(6):359–366.
204. Chiesa A, Serretti A. Mindfulness-based interventions for chronic pain: A systematic review of the evidence. *J Alternat Complement Med*. 2011;17(1):83–93.
205. Veehof MM, Trompetter H, Bohlmeijer ET, Schreurs K. Acceptance-and mindfulness-based interventions for the treatment of chronic pain: A meta-analytic review. *Cogn Behav Ther*. 2016;45(1):5–31.
206. Bawa FLM, Mercer SW, Atherton RJ, et al. Does mindfulness improve outcomes in patients with chronic pain? Systematic review and meta-analysis. *Br J Gen Pract*. 2015;65(635):e387–e400.
207. Cramer H, Lauche R, Paul A, Dobos G. Mindfulness-based stress reduction for breast cancer—a systematic review and meta-analysis. *Curr Oncol*. 2012;19(5):343–352.
208. Kroenke K, Baye F, Lourens SG, et al. Automated self-management (ASM) vs. ASM-enhanced collaborative care for chronic pain and mood symptoms: The CAMMPS randomized clinical trial. *J Gen Intern Med*. 2019;34:1806–1814.
209. Borsari B, Li Y, Tighe J, et al. A pilot trial of collaborative care with motivational interviewing to reduce opioid risk and improve chronic pain management. *Addiction*. 2021;116(9):2387–2397.
210. Thielke S, Corson K, Dobscha SK. Collaborative care for pain results in both symptom improvement and sustained reduction of pain and depression. *Gen Hosp Psychiatry*. 2015;37(2):139–143.
211. Kroenke K, Krebs EE, Wu J, Yu Z, Chumbler NR, Bair MJ. Telecare collaborative management of chronic pain in primary care: A randomized clinical trial. *JAMA*. 2014;312(3):240–248.
212. DeBar L, Mayhew M, Benes L, et al. A primary care–based cognitive behavioral therapy intervention for long-term opioid users with chronic pain: A randomized pragmatic trial. *Ann Intern Med*. 2022;175(1):46–55.
213. George MS, Nahas Z, Borckardt JJ, et al. Brain stimulation for the treatment of psychiatric disorders. *Curr Opin Psychiatry*. 2007;20(3):250–254.
214. Engels G, Francke AL, van Meijel B, et al. Clinical pain in schizophrenia: A systematic review. *J Pain*. 2014;15(5):457–467.

OTHER PSYCHIATRIC DISORDERS   115

215. Kishi T, Matsuda Y, Mukai T, et al. A cross-sectional survey to investigate the prevalence of pain in Japanese patients with major depressive disorder and schizophrenia. *Comprehens Psychiatry*. 2015;59:91–97.

216. Jochum T, Letzsch A, Greiner W, Wagner G, Sauer H, Bär K-J. Influence of antipsychotic medication on pain perception in schizophrenia. *Psychiatry Res*. 2006;142(2–3):151–156.

217. Guieu R, Samuelian J, Coulouvrat H. Objective evaluation of pain perception in patients with schizophrenia. *Br J Psychiatry*. 1994;164(2):253–255.

218. De la Fuente-Sandoval C, Favila R, Gómez-Martin D, Pellicer F, Graff-Guerrero A. Functional magnetic resonance imaging response to experimental pain in drug-free patients with schizophrenia. *Psychiatry Res Neuroimag*. 2010;183(2):99–104.

219. de la Fuente-Sandoval C, Favila R, Gómez-Martín D, León-Ortiz P, Graff-Guerrero A. Neural response to experimental heat pain in stable patients with schizophrenia. *J Psychiatric Res*. 2012;46(1):128–134.

220. Stubbs B, Thompson T, Acaster S, Vancampfort D, Gaughran F, Correll CU. Decreased pain sensitivity among people with schizophrenia: A meta-analysis of experimental pain induction studies. *Pain*. 2015;156(11):2121–2131.

221. Potvin S, Marchand S. Hypoalgesia in schizophrenia is independent of antipsychotic drugs: A systematic quantitative review of experimental studies. *Pain*. 2008;138(1):70–78.

222. Kim DJ, Mirmina J, Narine S, et al. Altered physical pain processing in different psychiatric conditions. *Neurosci Biobehav Rev*. 2022;133:104510.

223. Kuritzky A, Mazeh D, Levi A. Headache in schizophrenic patients: A controlled study. *Cephalalgia*. 1999;19(8):725–727.

224. De Hert M, Cohen D, Bobes J, et al. Physical illness in patients with severe mental disorders. II. Barriers to care, monitoring and treatment guidelines, plus recommendations at the system and individual level. *World Psychiatry*. 2011;10(2):138.

225. Watson G, Chandarana P, Merskey H. Relationships between pain and schizophrenia. *Br J Psychiatry*. 1981;138(1):33–36.

226. De Almeida JG, Braga PE, Neto FL, de Mattos Pimenta CA. Chronic pain and quality of life in schizophrenic patients. *Revista Brasileira de Psiquiatria*. 2013;35(1):13–20.

227. Abplanalp SJ, Mueser KT, Fulford D. The role of physical pain in global functioning of people with serious mental illness. *Schizophrenia Res*. 2020;222:423–428.

228. Stubbs B, Gardner-Sood P, Smith S, et al. Pain is independently associated with reduced health related quality of life in people with psychosis. *Psychiatry Res*. 2015;230(2):585–591.

229. Snow AL, Jr JLS. Assessment and treatment of persistent pain in persons with cognitive and communicative impairment. *J Clin Psychol*. 2006;62(11):1379–1387.

230. Bonnot O, Anderson GM, Cohen D, Willer JC, Tordjman S. Are patients with schizophrenia insensitive to pain? A reconsideration of the question. *Clin J Pain*. 2009;25(3):244–252.

231. Wells N, Pasero C, McCaffery M. Improving the quality of care through pain assessment and management. In: RG Hughes, ed. *Patient Safety and Quality: An Evidence-Based Handbook for Nurses*. Agency for Healthcare Research and Quality;2008: chapter 17.

232. Phelan M, Stradins L, Morrison S. Physical health of people with severe mental illness. *BMJ*. 2001 Feb 24;322(7284):443–444.

233. Dickerson FB, Brown CH, Daumit GL, et al. Health status of individuals with serious mental illness. *Schizophrenia Bull*. 2006;32(3):584–589.

234. Fleischhacker WW, Cetkovich-Bakmas M, De Hert M, et al. Comorbid somatic illnesses in patients with severe mental disorders: Clinical, policy, and research challenges. *J Clin Psychiatry*. 2008;69(4):514.

235. Heald A. Physical health in schizophrenia: A challenge for antipsychotic therapy. *Eur Psychiatry*. 2010;25:S6–S11.

236. Shin SW, Lee JS, Abdi S, Lee SJ, Kim KH. Antipsychotics for patients with pain. *Korean J Pain*. 2019;32(1):3–11.

116   MATTHEW J. BAIR AND ASHLI A. OWEN-SMITH

237. Visser E, Schug S. The role of ketamine in pain management. *Biomed Pharmacother.* 2006;60(7):341–348.

238. Oga K, Kojima T, Matsuura M, et al. Effects of low-dose ketamine on neuropathic pain: An electroencephalogram–electrooculogram/behavioral study. *Psychiatry Clin Neurosci.* 2002;56(4):355–363.

239. Benyamin RM, Vallejo R, Kramer J, Rafeyan R. Corticosteroid induced psychosis in the pain management setting. *Pain Physician.* 2008;11(6):917–920.

240. Tumenta T, Thanju A, Perera P, et al. Opioid-induced psychosis in a patient with sickle cell disease. *Cureus.* 2021;13(6):e15557.

241. Taylor MT, Horton DB, Juliano T, Olfson M, Gerhard T. Outpatient prescribing of opioids to adults diagnosed with mental disorders in the United States. *Drug Alcohol Depend.* 2021;219:108414.

242. Szmulewicz AG, Bateman BT, Levin R, Huybrechts KF. Risk of overdose associated with co-prescription of antipsychotics and opioids: A population-based cohort study. *Schizophrenia bull.* 2022;48(2):405–413.

243. Onwumere J, Stubbs B, Stirling M, et al. Pain management in people with severe mental illness: An agenda for progress. *Pain.* 2022;163(9):1653–1660.

244. Harris JI, Hanson D, Leskela J, et al. Reconsidering research exclusion for serious mental illness: Ethical principles, current status, and recommendations. *J Psychiatric Res.* 2021;143:138–143.

245. Cieślik B, Mazurek J, Rutkowski S, Kiper P, Turolla A, Szczepańska-Gieracha J. Virtual reality in psychiatric disorders: A systematic review of reviews. *Complement Ther Med.* 2020;52:102480.

246. Ju P, Zhao D, Zhu C, et al. Deep transcranial magnetic stimulation as a potential approach for digital pain management in patients with psychotic disorder. *Neurosci Bull.* 2023;39(1):89–93.

247. Otis JD, Keane TM, Kerns RD, Monson C, Scioli E. The development of an integrated treatment for veterans with comorbid chronic pain and posttraumatic stress disorder. *Pain Med.* 2009;10(7):1300–1311.

7

The Impact of Social and Structural Determinants on Depression, Prescription Opioid Use, Opioid Misuse, and Opioid Use Disorder

Fred Rottnek and Jennifer K. Bello-Kottenstette

7.1 Introduction

The immense impact of social and structural determinants of health (SSDOH) is well established, with the influence of personal and environmental factors—or the more traditional language of "nature and nurture"—on behavioral health being discussed for decades. Factors can be described as risks and protectors for development of substance use disorders (SUD) and mental illness. They exist in multiple systems, including in personal or familial relationships, communities, and society. These factors are correlated and cumulative.[1] In recent years, research has focused on questions related to the impact of SSDOH on interventions for prevention, diagnosis, treatment, and recovery support for people with SUDs.[2-7]

Alegria et al. describe the critical need to address the underappreciated role of social determinants to make mental health and addiction treatment effective, stating that "the price of hopelessness, emotional instability, and chronic uncertainty can only lead to poor behavioral health, taking away the opportunity for recovery."[8] The opioid overdose crisis is fueled by economic and social upheaval, with opioids being used as a refuge from physical and psychological trauma, concentrated disadvantage, isolation, and hopelessness.[5] In their literature review, Singh et al. identify multiple factors that contribute to disparities in the opioid epidemic related to drug overdoses, mortality, pain management, and treatment outcomes including lack of education and economic opportunities, poor working conditions, and low social

---

Fred Rottnek and Jennifer K. Bello-Kottenstette, *The Impact of Social and Structural Determinants on Depression, Prescription Opioid Use, Opioid Misuse, and Opioid Use Disorder* In: *Pain, the Opioid Epidemic, & Depression.* Edited by: Jeffrey F. Scherrer & Jane C. Ballantyne, Oxford University Press. © Oxford University Press 2024. DOI: 10.1093/9780197675250.003.0007

capital in disadvantaged communities.[9] In a recent scoping review, Park et al. propose a novel framework that incorporates social determinants in the foreground of the opioid epidemic.[10] They describe both micro- and macro-level social determinants that influence initiation of drug use including trauma and social exposure/access to prescription drugs and illicit drugs as well as structural racism, income inequality, and lack of affordable housing. Finally, in a review of qualitative studies on the progression from initial nonmedical prescription opioid use to use disorder, the most cited reasons for initiation and motivation for continued use are a response to life stressors including as a means of self-medicating psychological issues, effects of trauma, or emotional pain.[11]

Healthy People 2030 is a program of the U.S. Department of Health and Human Services that has promoted data-driven national objectives to improve health and well-being over the course of a specified decade. Healthy People defines social determinants of health (SDOH) as conditions in the environment where people are born, live, work, play, worship, and age that affect a wide range of health, function, and quality of life outcomes and risks.[12] Healthy People groups SDOH into five domains: economic stability, education access and quality, healthcare access and quality, neighborhood and built environment, and social and community context (see Figure 7.1).

7.2 Impact of Economic Stability

Economic stability includes adequacy and nature of employment, income stability and poverty, housing stability and quality of housing, and food security with access to healthy food. Poverty and financial insecurity contribute to the development and exacerbation of toxic stress, chronic disease, and other poor mental and physical health outcomes.[13] Improving economic stability has been linked to children's scholastic achievement and academic attainment.[14]

Housing is the largest budget item for most families, and lack of economic stability exacerbates related housing security. Basic housing is the foundation for protection from the environment and access to water, food, clothing, and other basic necessities—including human connection and psychological well-being.[15] Low-quality housing results in a variety of poor health conditions, including asthma, lead poisoning, developmental delays, and exposure to communicable diseases.[16,17] These physical problems can lead to additional behavioral problems in youth and young adults, such as anger,

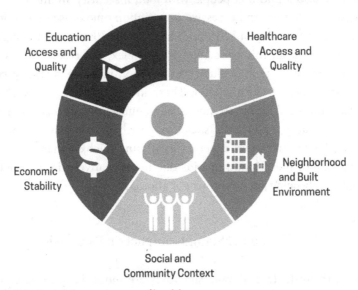

Figure 7.1 Social determinants of health.
Source: Healthy People 2030, U.S. Department of Health and Human Services, Office of Disease Prevention and Health Promotion. https://health.gov/healthypeople/objectives-and-data/social-determinants-health. Accessed Mar. 2, 2023.

depression, and anxiety. The entire family can have increased anxiety and depression from inadequate heat, dampness, noise, and disrepair. Evictions and other housing disruptions exacerbate negative outcomes listed above.[18]

7.2.1 Economic Stability Impact on Pain

People with unstable economic situations are more likely to develop chronic pain, develop dependence on analgesic medications, and have greater challenges to gaining and maintaining employment. At the same time, co-occurring mental illness and chronic pain are associated with work disability.[19] Improvement of functioning is most effective when rehabilitation programs address activities related to both work and employment in addition to other areas of life outside of occupational settings.[20]

Food insecurity, in particular, has been identified as a powerful indicator of chronic pain. In an analysis of the population representative Canadian Community Health Survey, Men et al. found that, compared to people who are food secure, people experiencing food insecurity are more likely to experience severe pain and pain-related restrictions in activities.[21] Other researchers also found that people with food insecurity are more likely to demonstrate intensive and excessive prescription opioid use in addition to acquiring and using opioids through means other than medical prescription. The reasons for this association are complex, and risk factors that are more prevalent among individuals who are food-insecure likely contribute to the experience of chronic pain. These include chronic stress, chronic physical and mental illness, strenuous labor, nutrient inadequacy, abnormal weight, poor sleep, and lack of social support.[22-25] These risk factors may lead to prolonged and severe experiences of pain, which could influence possible overuse of prescription opioids due to alternative pain management strategies likely being less convenient or affordable.[26]

7.2.2 Economic Stability Impact on Depression

People with unstable economic situations are more likely to have worse outcomes with depression and other mental illness, and these conditions more negatively impact their quality of life.[27,28] Housing insecurity is correlated with a high incidence of maternal depression and other mental health concerns in the family.[29] Other correlations in housing-insecure individuals and families include trauma and lack of ready access to medical care, which can further exacerbate depression. Limitations of health professional capacity and skill in treating patients with psychosocial conditions further limits care.[30] Conversely, current studies suggest that employment, as well as rehabilitative counseling and human resource policies, can enhance resiliency against depression.[31]

7.2.3 Economic Stability Impact on Opioid Use Disorder

People with economic insecurity are more likely to have opioid use disorder (OUD) arising from both illicit and prescribed opioids,[32] particularly when this insecurity is manifest in housing insecurity. The correlation between housing insecurity and OUD is strong and poses challenges to treatment and retention in recovery programs.[33] People with economic insecurity who are unhoused often have little to no social support network, and finding food and shelter takes top priority over participating in recovery programs. Finally, OUD co-occurrence among people who are housing-insecure with a co-occurring diagnosis of bipolar disorder and schizophrenia is particularly high.[34]

A housing-first model for people with OUD has gained recognition as an approach to help people achieve safety so that treatment can occur.[33,35] Other recognized recovery elements are vocational and financial services, with employment being one of the strongest predictors of positive outcomes for people with SUD.[36] Vocational services within recovery programs can help people with OUD overcome the numerous internal and external barriers to finding work, such as lack of vocational training and education deficits, unrealistic expectations for employment, limited opportunities, and employer bias.[37] Finally, barriers to financial wellness experienced by individuals with mental health and substance use issues include limited income, poor credit, and minimal access to financial institutions. These barriers limit further economic opportunity and need to be addressed in the course of treatment.[38]

7.3 Impact of Education Access and Quality

Education access and quality enhances an individual's ability to gain knowledge and behavior that is central to thriving. High school completion is seen as the minimum level of education needed for success in adulthood. Completion of high school is strongly associated with employment status, income, and health.[39] Likewise, completing some amount of college has protective and health-promoting effects, with the greatest effects experienced by individuals who started off with the least educational access and resources.[40]

In addition to formal education, both health and financial literacy are needed skills for thriving. Health literacy is defined by Healthy People and the U.S. Department of Health and Human Services as (a) *personal health literacy*, an individual's capacity to find, understand, and use information and services to inform health-related decisions, and (b) *organizational health literacy*, the degree to which organizations equitably enable individuals to find, understand, and use information and services to inform health-related decisions and actions.[41] Low personal health literacy is a social risk that is associated with worse healthcare and outcomes. Organizational health literacy is a social determinant of health because living in a community where healthcare organizations lack organizational health literacy can negatively affect the quality of care delivered and, as a result, health outcomes.

Finally, financial literacy, which is the set of skills and knowledge needed for people to make informed decisions about their finances, also has

122 FRED ROTTNEK AND JENNIFER K. BELLO-KOTTENSTETTE

implications for healthcare behaviors. This is due to changes in healthcare delivery models that shift more healthcare costs to patients, leading to greater patient financial responsibilities.[42,43]

7.3.1 Education Access and Quality: Impact on Pain

Chronic pain in youth and adolescents has both immediate and long-term impact on educational, vocational, and social outcomes.[44] For example, youth reporting chronic pain tend to report more educational disruptions, lower educational attainment, and lower financial and occupational status. They also report lower-quality romantic relationships and a higher likelihood of having biological children early in adulthood. A recent study using nationally representative survey data of 30 to 49-year-old adults from 2010 to 2017 found a complex relationship between educational attainment and pain.[45] Zajacova and co-authors found that, compared to adults with a high school degree, having less than a high school degree was associated with a higher odds of reporting pain, while bachelor's and postgraduate levels were associated with a lower odds of pain. These associations were no longer statistically significant when controlling for sex, race/ethnicity, and age group. Interestingly, adults with a general education diploma (GED) and those with some college but no degree experienced higher odds of pain than those with a high school degree in both unadjusted and adjusted models, with results varying by sex, race/ethnicity, and age group.[45]

7.3.2 Education Access and Quality Impact on Depression

Higher education has a protective effect on the development and progression of major depression.[46] For people with psychiatric disabilities, financial education can actually improve quality of life and overall functioning.[43,47]

7.3.3 Education Access and Quality Impact on Opioid Use Disorder

Death from opioid overdose disproportionally impacts people with numerous indicators of low socioeconomic status, including education level.

SOCIAL AND STRUCTURAL DETERMINANTS   123

Multiple studies have found higher levels of educational attainment associated with lower rates of opioid-related fatal overdose.[48,49] Ellis et al. found
that, compared to the general population, patients entering treatment for
OUD were less likely to have earned an advanced degree.[50] In addition, the
majority of respondents indicated that opioid use negatively impacted their
education.

OUD educational programs regarding awareness, prevention, and harm
reduction are evidence-based and have been utilized, albeit underutilized,
for decades.[51] While these programs have been historically underutilized,
they are carried out in a variety of formats, including in a formal educational
setting, an informal community setting, and in the home, and have long-
term positive benefit in mitigating development of SUD.[52-54] Educational
and prevention programs are also available for adults and seniors who may
be at greater risk for OUD. These programs have been shown to decrease
opioid misuse, overdose, and diversion.[55-57]

7.4 Impact of Healthcare Access and Quality

Healthcare access and quality involves the ability of the individual to access
needed services and the capacity of the system to deliver these services in
a timely, high-quality, and coordinated way. In the United States, access to
health coverage and/or insurance complicates this process. While studies
have demonstrated that people, particularly children and youth, benefit
from insurance, there is still lack of consensus in the United States about
who is responsible for providing what level of coverage.[58,59] Varying levels of
health insurance coverage lead to inconsistent access to screening, diagnosis,
and treatment modalities.[60,61] Access and capacity are further hampered by
professional workforce shortages.

7.4.1 Health Care Access and Quality Impact on
Acute and Chronic Pain

Access to the full range of services needed for people with chronic pain has
been difficult in the United States, even for patients with relatively generous
employer-based insurance. Some of the reasons for limited access to effective services have remained relatively constant over decades, including lack

of pain specialists, inadequate pain studies, and inadequate compensation for non-pharmaceutical treatment of pain.[62] Other interventions, particularly the use of opioid medications, have been on a wide-ranging pendulum swing of availability, professional messaging, and regulations. And while some standardization is emerging with the first clinical practice guidelines issued by the U.S. Centers for Disease Control (CDC) and recently updated CDC guidelines for prescribing opioids for pain, there remains inconsistent implementation of guidelines among medical practices and healthcare systems.[63,64]

However, decades of literature exists showing that the gold standard for effective management of chronic pain is patient-centered interprofessional collaborative practice teams.[65] These interprofessional teams are effective because they recognize and address the multifactorial contributions to the development and treatment of chronic pain. However, funding such programs has always been problematic due to the time, intensity, and interprofessional nature of the work, along with the need to train health professional learners in interprofessional team-based care.[64,66] In an analysis of 2017 Essential Health Benefits benchmark plans across all states, Bonakdar and co-authors found that insurance coverage actually discourages multidisciplinary rehabilitation for chronic pain management by providing vague guidelines, restricting ongoing treatments, and excluding behavioral or complementary therapy despite known benefits.[67] Finally, comprehensive pain management services may not be available to those most in need due to inequitable health insurance coverage and practical access to such services.

7.4.2 Health Care Access and Quality Impact on Depression

People with depression do better with access to medication as well as psychotherapy, exercise, and other treatment modalities. While some people have success with medical therapy, others do better with non-medication therapy and some do better with a combination of interventions.[68,69] Importantly, patients with both OUD and co-occurring depression fare better with medication treatment of both conditions.[70] Despite the well-established benefits of various forms of treatment, the availability of trained healthcare professionals to treat depression and OUD limits access and capacity for care.[71,72]

7.4.3 Healthcare Access and Quality Impact on Opioid Use Disorder

While copious studies have been published on the efficacy of medications approved by the U.S. Food and Drug Administration (FDA) (methadone, buprenorphine, and naltrexone oral and long-acting injectable formulations) to treat OUD and prevent relapse,[73] there remain almost as many barriers to care for people seeking services.[74] These barriers include the workforce capacity of not only the prescribing providers but also all the professionals needed to provide evidence-based OUD treatment and recovery support. The stigma associated with harm reduction and treatment services is still pervasive in traditional healthcare systems.[75]

Education and advocacy throughout the treatment continuum are needed to address the lack of treatment and the inequality of provision in such treatment.[76] While laws and regulations were modified or suspended during the COVID-19 public health emergency, it is still unclear what rules may snap back into place and what will be extended or permanently changed. Virtual healthcare has allowed many people access to OUD treatment in ways that traditional in-person care did not allow.[77-79] Suspension of the Ryan-Haight Act and other interstate limitations in license reciprocities also allow greater access to care—especially to populations limited by geography, transportation, or local provider availability. Additional innovation has also produced novel mobile prevention, harm reduction, and treatment units, which have brought services to rural areas, treatment deserts, and other hard-to-reach populations. These changes facilitated creative and effective innovation in delivery of low-barrier OUD treatment services.[80-82]

7.5 Impact of Neighborhood and Built Environment

Neighborhood and built environment include structures, infrastructure, and activities within a community, including transportation, utilities, pollution, violence, abuse, neglect, and the associated toxicities. The ability of an individual and a family unit to thrive within their neighborhood and built environment is key to health and well-being. While assets and needs vary among rural, suburban, and urban environments, all share qualities that promote health as well as opportunities to maximize health.

Environmental conditions include safe water and air and minimal exposures to unhealthy conditions and hazardous waste.[83] A healthy environment is one where trauma, neglect, and violence—including toxic stress and trauma—is minimized or absent.[84] The "Pair of ACES" is one of the commonly used models which links negative childhood and adult health conditions to both adverse childhood experiences and adverse community experiences.[85–89]

Health-promoting environments have accessible and free or affordable transportation for individuals to participate in societal functions and access healthcare and health-promoting behaviors.[90–93] Healthy behaviors are also supported with access to wireless phone networks and wi-fi coverage. With these technologies, individuals are able to participate in life, work, and occupations; access medical care; and participate in society.[94]

7.5.1 Neighborhood and Environment Impact on Pain

Where people live, including rural, suburban, and urban environments, affects how they perceive pain, cope with pain, and seek treatment for pain. The long-term impact of pain also depends on people's environments. A North Carolina study, conducted in that state with great diversity in rural, suburban, and urban residence, found that chronic pain is more often reported among rural and suburban residents.[95] The built environment of treatment locations also has the ability to impact a person's perception of pain. These factors include light and access to nature as well as nature sounds and images, either naturally or through video or virtual reality.[96]

7.5.2 Neighborhood and Environment Impact on Depression

The home environment of a person, particularly a young person, includes their relationships within the home—both positive, nurturing relationships and neglect, abuse, and other forms of trauma. These latter conditions have the ability to alter children's physiological function and development, resulting in poor physical and emotional health as adults.[97] Anderson and co-authors found that, among 2,000 participants in a longitudinal study of cardiovascular risk factors in the rural south, built environment measured using neighborhood scales that included the domains of path, pedestrian safety, aesthetics, commercial and civic destinations, physical security,

SOCIAL AND STRUCTURAL DETERMINANTS   127

and land use, was associated with both the prevalence and risk of depression, with stronger associations in neighborhoods with higher poverty.[98] In a cross-sectional analysis from a population-representative sample in the Netherlands, perceived social environment was found to play a role in depression severity, independent of sociodemographics, with neighborhood social cohesion, pleasantness, and safety being associated with lower depressive symptoms and perceived distance to green space and traffic correlated with increased severity.[99] Finally, safe, accessible outdoor environments for relaxation and exercise,[100] including parks and other green spaces, are associated with improved mental health.[101] The great, uncontrolled public health experiment of COVID-19 reinforced these findings.

7.5.3 Neighborhood and Environment Impact on Opioid Use Disorder

People, particularly youth, with access to safe environments and neighbors have natural protection against the development of OUD.[102] The nature of an individual, a family, and the community provides an interconnected set of both protective factors and risk factors for development of SUDs, including OUDs. Individual risk factors described by Nawi and co-authors include high impulsivity, rebelliousness, impairment of emotional self-regulation, experience of trauma, co-occurring mental illness, low perceived risk, and easy access to drugs.[102] Family risk factors described by Nawi and co-authors include low supervision of children, uncontrolled pocket money, and presence of substance-using family members. Community risk factors include the presence of peers who use drugs.[102]

7.6 Impact of Social and Community Context and Connectedness

Connection to others is necessary for thriving. Weakening and dissolution of the roles and responsibilities that facilitate connection has been documented among White and rural populations in recent years—a phenomenon that has been termed "deaths of despair."[103–105] These deaths include suicide, poisonings and overdoses, and alcohol-related liver disease.[106] However, social participation has been strained or denied since the nation's founding through institutional racism, stigma, and bias toward Black, Indigenous, and people of color (BIPOC) and other minorities, such as the LGBTQ and transgender populations.[18,107-109] This discrimination has impacted other SSDOH mentioned throughout this chapter, but it has also contributed to the growth of the institutional criminal legal system in the United States in which BIPOC and other minority populations have been disproportionately negatively affected.[110-113]

Social media use is a more recent social phenomenon, with both positive and negative impacts. While those using social media report it as a means of connecting with others and broadening one's perspective, it can also be used to foment separation and polarization within society.[114,115]

7.6.1 Social, Community Context, and Connectedness Impact on Pain

Social cohesion and strength of a social network appear to impact how people understand and cope with chronic pain. For example, in a cross-sectional personal network analysis of 600 relationships, authors found that both emotional and instrumental support are highly valued and necessary for patients with chronic pain.[116] Perceptions of how one is viewed in society and how that impacts pain treatment also impacts perception of pain and treatment of pain, with higher levels of perceived injustice found to be associated with heightened daily levels of opioid craving that are mediated by catastrophizing, or imagining the worst possible outcome.[117]

Sullivan and Ballantyne describe the interaction between social and physical pain and the need to understand the social aspects of chronic pain in order to improve treatment approaches.[118] The experience of stress and social isolation in the form of social rejection that involves intentional separation of important social bonds is one of the strongest risk factors for both depression and disruption of the opioid system. The impact of repeated or extreme stress on the endogenous opioid system may contribute to social isolation in addition to both chronic pain and risk for developing addiction.

7.6.2 Social, Community Context, and Connectedness Impact on Depression

Likewise, social cohesion and strength of a social network impact how people understand and cope with depression. This connection has been demonstrated among youth with the social cohesion factors defined as safety, trust, positive social connections, helping others, and a lack of crime and violence.[119] The lack of social cohesion and a strong social network has also been explored among older adults. Lack of community and neighborhood cohesion results in a higher rate of depression.[120] Furthermore, in situations of community-wide natural disasters, social cohesion is protective against depression.[121]

Among BIPOC and other minorities, protective mechanisms against depression have been identified. In a review of 39 studies, researchers identified the protective factors of employment, extracurricular activities, father–adolescent closeness, familism, maternal support, attending predominately minority schools, neighborhood composition, non-parent support, parental inductive reasoning, religiosity, self-esteem, social activities, and positive early teacher relationships.[122]

7.6.3 Social, Community Context, and Connectedness Impact on Opioid Use Disorder

SUDs are often called diseases of disconnection. One central principle of most models of recovery is reconnection with self and others. This importance of connection for a person with SUD to a community is recognized in programs as diverse as treatment courts[123] and peer recovery support,[124,125] and by treating clinicians.[126] For indigenous cultures, this reconnection can come with incorporation of traditional healing practices into treatment services.[127] Finally, COVID-19 stressed society, generating isolation and disconnection. SUD patterns, including OUD prevalence and record opioid overdose rates during the pandemic, reinforced this principle.[128,129]

7.7 Conclusion

The impact of social and structural determinants of health on pain, depression, chronic or problematic opioid use, and development of OUD have been well established in recent decades. Movements, such as Thriving Together: A Springboard for Equitable Recovery and Resilience in Communities Across America, seek to define resources communities need to organize in order to thrive.[130] It is a community-driven model that offers hope for overcoming those structural and social determinants of health that lead to health disparities. Yet there are few studies of social and structural determinants of health and the co-occurring comorbidities of pain, depression, and OUD. An understanding of the interconnectedness of co-occurring pain, depression, and OUD and the public health drivers of this interconnectedness is essential to truly address these complex problems at patient, family, and community levels. A multilevel and interdisciplinary approach that extends beyond a traditional healthcare model, and even beyond a social and structural determinants of health model, is needed to move upstream to prevent these comorbidities. Such an approach has been coined "political determinants of health." In Daniel Dawes own words, "The political determinants of health involve the systematic process of structuring relationships, distributing resources, and administering power, operating simultaneously in ways that mutually reinforce or influence one another to shape opportunities that either advance health equity or exacerbate health inequities."[131] Just as development of chronic pain, depression, and OUD is interconnected in initiation, diagnosis, and treatment, prevention education and implementation require an understanding of the multifactorial drivers of these conditions.

References

1. Substance Abuse and Mental Health Services Administration. Risk and protective factors. 2019. https://www.samhsa.gov/sites/default/files/20190718-samhsa-risk-protective-factors.pdf. Accessed Mar. 1, 2023.
2. Bierut LJ. Genetic vulnerability and susceptibility to substance dependence. *Neuron.* 2011;69(4):618–627.
3. El-Bassel N, Shoptaw S, Goodman-Meza D, Ono H. Addressing long overdue social and structural determinants of the opioid epidemic. *Drug Alcohol Depend* 2021;222:108679.
4. Hansen H, Jordan A, Plough A, Alegria M, Cunningham C, Ostrovsky A. Lessons for the opioid crisis-integrating social determinants of health into clinical care. *Am J Public Health.* 2022;112(S2):S109–S111.
5. Dasgupta N, Beletsky L, Ciccarone D. Opioid crisis: No easy fix to its social and economic determinants. *Am J Public Health.* 2018;108(2):182–186.
6. Butkus R, Rapp K, Cooney TG, Engel LS. Envisioning a better U.S. health care system for all: Reducing barriers to care and addressing social determinants of health. *Ann Intern Med.* 2020;172(2 Suppl):S50–S59.
7. Humphreys K, Shover CL, Andrews CM, et al. Responding to the opioid crisis in North America and beyond: Recommendations of the Stanford-Lancet Commission. *Lancet.* 2022;399(10324):555–604.
8. Alegría M, Frank RG, Hansen HB, Sharfstein JM, Shim RS, Tierney M. Transforming mental health and addiction services. *Health Aff (Project Hope).* 2021;40(2):226–234.
9. Singh GK, Kim IE, Girmay M, et al. Opioid epidemic in the United States: Empirical trends, and a literature review of social determinants and epidemiological, pain management, and treatment patterns. *Int J MCH AIDS.* 2019;8(2):89–100.
10. Park JN, Rouhani S, Beletsky L, Vincent L, Saloner B, Sherman SG. Situating the continuum of overdose risk in the social determinants of health: A new conceptual framework. *Milbank Q.* 2020;98(3):700–746.

SOCIAL AND STRUCTURAL DETERMINANTS 131

11. Cicero TJ, Ellis MS. The prescription opioid epidemic: A review of qualitative studies on the progression from initial use to abuse. *Dialogues Clin Neurosci.* 2017;19(3):259–269.

12. Office of Disease Prevention and Health Promotion. Healthy People 2030: Social determinants of health. U.S. Department of Health and Human Services. https://health.gov/healthypeople/objectives-and-data/social-determinants-health. 2020. Accessed Dec. 19, 2022.

13. Well Being Trust. Meaningful work & wealth. https://thriving.us/vital-conditions/meaningful-work-wealth/. 2023. Accessed Mar. 3, 2023.

14. Duncan GJ, Magnuson K, Votruba-Drzal E. Moving beyond correlations in assessing the consequences of poverty. *Annu Rev Psychol.* 2017;68:413–434.

15. Jacobs DE. Environmental health disparities in housing. *Am J Public Health.* 2011;101 (Suppl 1):S115–S122.

16. Gold AE. No home for justice: How eviction perpetuates health inequity among low-income and minority tenants among low-income and minority tenants. *Georgetown Journal on Poverty Law and Policy.* 2016;24.

17. Centers for Disease Control and Prevention. Children's environmental health. National Environmental Public Health Tracking Web site. https://www.cdc.gov/nceh/tracking/topics/ChildrensEnvironmentalHealth.htm Published 2022. Accessed Mar. 2, 2023.

18. Bradford AC, Bradford WD. The effect of evictions on accidental drug and alcohol mortality. *Health Serv Res.* 2020;55(1):9–17.

19. Braden JB, Zhang L, Zimmerman FJ, Sullivan MD. Employment outcomes of persons with a mental disorder and comorbid chronic pain. *Psychiatric Serv (Washington, DC).* 2008;59(8):878–885.

20. Friedli T, Gantschnig BE. The role of contextual factors on participation in the life area of work and employment after rehabilitation: A qualitative study on the views of persons with chronic pain. *Work.* 2022;71(1):119–132.

21. Men F, Fischer B, Urquia ML, Tarasuk V. Food insecurity, chronic pain, and use of prescription opioids. *SSM Popul Health.* 2021;14:100768.

22. Arenas DJ, Thomas A, Wang J, DeLisser HM. A systematic review and meta-analysis of depression, anxiety, and sleep disorders in US adults with food insecurity. *J Gen Intern Med.* 2019;34(12):2874–2882.

23. Kirkpatrick SI, Dodd KW, Parsons R, Ng C, Garriguet D, Tarasuk V. Household food insecurity is a stronger marker of adequacy of nutrient intakes among Canadian compared to American youth and adults. *J Nutr.* 2015;145(7):1596–1603.

24. Vozoris NT, Tarasuk VS. Household food insufficiency is associated with poorer health. *J Nutr.* 2003;133(1):120–126.

25. Martin MS, Maddocks E, Chen Y, Gilman SE, Colman I. Food insecurity and mental illness: disproportionate impacts in the context of perceived stress and social isolation. *Public Health.* 2016;132:86–91.

26. Bartram M, Stewart JM. Income-based inequities in access to psychotherapy and other mental health services in Canada and Australia. *Health Policy.* 2019;123(1):45–50.

27. DeCarlo Santiago C, Wadsworth ME, Stump J. Socioeconomic status, neighborhood disadvantage, and poverty-related stress: Prospective effects on psychological syndromes among diverse low-income families. *J Econ Psychol.* 2011;32(2):218–230.

28. Ridley M, Rao G, Schilbach F, Patel V. Poverty, depression, and anxiety: Causal evidence and mechanisms. *Science.* 2020;370(6522):eaay0214.

29. McGovern ME, Rokicki S, Reichman NE. Maternal depression and economic well-being: A quasi-experimental approach. *Soc Sci Med (1982).* 2022;305:115017.

30. Grant R, Gracy D, Goldsmith G, Shapiro A, Redlener IE. Twenty-five years of child and family homelessness: Where are we now? *Am J Public Health.* 2013;103(Suppl 2):e1–e10.

31. Heinz AJ, Meffert BN, Halvorson MA, Blonigen D, Timko C, Cronkite R. Employment characteristics, work environment, and the course of depression over 23 years: Does employment help foster resilience? *Depression Anxiety.* 2018;35(9):861–867.

32. Cicero TJ, Ellis MS, Surratt HL, Kurtz SP. The changing face of heroin use in the United States: A retrospective analysis of the past 50 years. *JAMA Psychiatry*. 2014;71(7):821–826.

33. Substance Abuse and Mental Health Services Administration. Whole-person care for people experiencing homelessness and opioid use disorder: A toolkit. 2021. https://nhchc.org/wp-content/uploads/2021/09/Homelessness_OUD_Toolkit_Part_I_Aug2021.pdf Accessed Feb. 23, 2023.

34. Ali MM, Sutherland H, Rosenoff E. Comorbid health conditions and treatment utilization among individuals with opioid use disorder experiencing homelessness. *Subst Use Misuse*. 2021;56(4):571–574.

35. Substance Abuse and Mental Health Services Administration. Recovery housing: Best practices and suggested guidelines. 2018. https://www.samhsa.gov/sites/default/files/housing-best-practices-100819.pdf. Accessed Feb. 23, 2023.

36. Magura S, Marshall T. The effectiveness of interventions intended to improve employment outcomes for persons with substance use disorder: An updated systematic review. *Subst Use Misuse*. 2020;55(13):2230–2236.

37. Substance Abuse and Mental Health Services Administration. Integrating vocational services into substance use disorder treatment. 2021. https://store.samhsa.gov/sites/default/files/SAMHSA_Digital_Download/pep20-02-01-019.pdf. Accessed Feb. 23, 2023.

38. Center on Integrated Health Care and Self-Directed Recovery. Building financial wellness. 2019. https://www.center4healthandsdc.org/building-financial-wellness.html. Accessed Feb. 23, 2023.

39. Qu S, Chattopadhyay SK, Hahn RA. High school completion programs: A community guide systematic economic review. *J Public Health Manag Pract*. 2016;22(3):E47–56.

40. Schafer MH, Wilkinson LR, Ferraro KF. Childhood (mis)fortune, educational attainment, and adult health: Contingent benefits of a college degree? *Soc Forces*. 2013;91(3):1007–1034.

41. Office of Disease Prevention and Health Promotion. Health literacy. U.S. Department of Health and Human Services. Healthy People 2030 Web site. https://health.gov/healthypeople/priority-areas/social-determinants-health/literature-summaries/health-literacy. Accessed Feb. 23, 2023.

42. Meyer M. Is financial literacy a determinant of health? *Patient*. 2017;10(4):381–387.

43. Patel MR, Kruger DJ, Cupal S, Zimmerman MA. Effect of financial stress and positive financial behaviors on cost-related nonadherence to health regimens among adults in a community-based setting. *Prevent Chronic Dis*. 2016;13:E46.

44. Murray CB, Groenewald CB, de la Vega R, Palermo TM. Long-term impact of adolescent chronic pain on young adult educational, vocational, and social outcomes. *Pain*. 2020;161(2):439–445.

45. Zajacova A, Rogers RG, Grodsky E, Grol-Prokopczyk H. The relationship between education and pain among adults aged 30–49 in the United States. *J Pain*. 2020;21(11-12):1270–1280.

46. Bauldry S. Variation in the protective effect of higher education against depression. *Society Mental Health*. 2015;5(2):145–161.

47. Cook JA, Burke JK, Petersen CA. Assessing the financial planning needs of Americans with mental illness. A report by the University of Illinois at Chicago Center on Mental Health Services Research and Policy. 2004. http://www.cmhsrp.uic.edu/download/CMHSRP_NEFE_Report.pdf. Accessed Feb. 24, 2023.

48. van Draanen J, Tsang C, Mitra S, Karamouzian M, Richardson L. Socioeconomic marginalization and opioid-related overdose: A systematic review. *Drug Alcohol Depend*. 2020;214:108127.

49. Altekruse SF, Cosgrove CM, Altekruse WC, Jenkins RA, Blanco C. Socioeconomic risk factors for fatal opioid overdoses in the United States: Findings from the Mortality Disparities in American Communities Study (MDAC). *PLoS One*. 2020;15(1):e0227966.

50. Ellis MS, Kasper ZA, Cicero TJ. The impact of opioid use disorder on levels of educational attainment: Perceived benefits and consequences. *Drug Alcohol Depend.* 2020;206:107618.
51. Horn KA, Pack RP, Trestman R, Lawson G. Almost everything we need to better serve children of the opioid crisis we learned in the 80s and 90s. *Front Public Health.* 2018;6:289.
52. Binswanger IA, Glanz JM. Pharmaceutical opioids in the home and youth: Implications for adult medical practice. *Subst Abuse.* 2015;36(2):141–143.
53. Volkow ND, Wargo EM. Association of severity of adolescent substance use disorders and long-term outcomes. *JAMA Netw Open.* 2022;5(4):e225656.
54. Markiewicz J, Swanberg K, Weis M. Awareness, education, and collaboration: Promising School-based opioid prevention approaches. Issue Brief: Project Aware. n.d. Accessed Feb. 24, 2023.
55. Substance Abuse and Mental Health Services Administration. Substance use disorders recovery with a focus on employment and education. 2021. https://store.samhsa.gov/sites/default/files/SAMHSA_Digital_Download/pep21-pl-guide-6.pdf. Accessed Mar. 2, 2023.
56. Rafa A. Education policy responses to the opioid crisis. 2019. https://www.ecs.org/wp-content/uploads/Education-Policy-Responses-to-the-Opioid-Crisis.pdf. Accessed Mar. 2, 2023.
57. National Council on Aging. The impact of the opioid epidemic on the aging services network and the older adults they serve. https://www.ncoa.org/article/the-impact-of-the-opioid-epidemic-on-the-aging-services-network-and-the-older-adults-they-serve. 2019. Accessed Mar. 2, 2023.
58. Murphey D. Health insurance coverage improves child well-being. 2017. https://www.childtrends.org/wp-content/uploads/2017/05/2017-22HealthInsurance_finalupdate.pdf. Accessed Feb. 24, 2023.
59. Georgetown University Health Policy Institute Center for Children and Families. Medicaid expansion: Good for parents and children. 2014. http://ccf.georgetown.edu/wp-content/uploads/2013/12/Expanding-Coverage-for-Parents-Helps-Children-2013.pdf.
60. Demeke HB, Merali S, Marks S, et al. Trends in use of telehealth among health centers during the COVID-19 pandemic – United States, June 26–November 6, 2020. *MMWR Morb Mortal Wkly Rep.* 2021;70(7):240–244.
61. Centers for Disease Control and Prevention. Telehealth and telemedicine. Public Health Professionals Gateway: Public Health Law Web site. https://www.cdc.gov/phlp/publications/topic/telehealth.html. 2020. Accessed Feb. 24, 2023.
62. AMA Pain Care Task Force. Addressing obstacles to evidence-informed pain care. *AMA J Ethics.* 2020;22(1):E709–717.
63. Dowell D, Haegerich TM, Chou R. CDC Guideline for prescribing opioids for chronic pain – United States, 2016. MMWR recommendations and reports. *Morb Mortal Weekly Rep.* 2016;65(1):1–49.
64. Dowell D, Ragan KR, Jones CM, Baldwin GT, Chou R. CDC Clinical practice guideline for prescribing opioids for pain – United States, 2022. MMWR recommendations and reports. *Morb Mortal Weekly Rep.* 2022;71(3):1–95.
65. Gordon DB, Watt-Watson J, Hogans BB. Interprofessional pain education: With, from, and about competent, collaborative practice teams to transform pain care. *Pain Rep.* 2018;3(3):e663.
66. Block L, Lalley A, LaVine NA, et al. The financial cost of interprofessional ambulatory training: What's the bottom line? *J Grad Med Educ.* 2021;13(1):108–112.
67. Bonakdar R, Palanker D, Sweeney MM. Analysis of state insurance coverage for nonpharmacologic treatment of low back pain as recommended by the American College of Physicians Guidelines. *Glob Adv Health Med.* 2019;8:2164956119855629.
68. Gelenberg AJ, Freeman MP, Markowitz JC, et al. Practice guideline for the treatment of patients with major depressive disorder. 2010. https://psychiatryonline.org/pb/assets/raw/sitewide/practice_guidelines/guidelines/mdd.pdf. Accessed Feb. 27, 2023.

69. Cipriani A, Furukawa TA, Salanti G, et al. Comparative efficacy and acceptability of 21 antidepressant drugs for the acute treatment of adults with major depressive disorder: A systematic review and network meta-analysis. *Lancet.* 2018;391(10128):1357–1366.
70. Zhang K, Jones CM, Compton WM, Guy GP, Evans ME, Volkow ND. Association between receipt of antidepressants and retention in buprenorphine treatment for opioid use disorder: A population-based retrospective cohort study. *J Clin Psychiatry.* 2022;83(3):21m14001.
71. Covino NA. Developing the behavioral health workforce: Lessons from the States. *Adm Policy Ment Health.* 2019;46(6):689–695.
72. University of Michigan School of Public Health. Behavioral health workforce research center. https://www.behavioralhealthworkforce.org/. 2016. Accessed Feb. 27, 2023.
73. Lagisetty P, Klasa K, Bush C, Heisler M, Chopra V, Bohnert A. Primary care models for treating opioid use disorders: What actually works? A systematic review. *PLoS One.* 2017;12(10):e0186315.
74. Mackey K, Veazie S, Anderson J, Bourne D, Peterson K. Barriers and facilitators to the use of medications for opioid use disorder: A rapid review. *J Gen Intern Med.* 2020;35(Suppl 3):954–963.
75. FXB Center for Health & Human Rights at Harvard University. From the War on Drugs to harm reduction: Imagining a just overdose crisis response. 2020. https://cdn1.sph.harv ard.edu/wp-content/uploads/sites/2464/2020/12/Opioid-Whitepaper-Final-12-2020. pdf. Accessed Feb. 27, 2023.
76. National Association of County and City Health Officials. Opioid epidemic toolkit. 2021. https://www.naccho.org/programs/community-health/injury-and-violence/opioid-epidemic/local-health-departments-and-the-opioid-epidemic-a-toolkit#prevention. 2023. Accessed Feb. 27, 2023.
77. Mattocks KM, Moore DT, Wischik DL, Lazar CM, Rosen MI. Understanding opportunities and challenges with telemedicine-delivered buprenorphine during the COVID-19 pandemic. *J Subst Abuse Treat.* 2022;139:108777.
78. Lockard R, Priest KC, Gregg J, Buchheit BM. A qualitative study of patient experiences with telemedicine opioid use disorder treatment during COVID-19. *Subst Abuse.* 2022;43(1):1150–1157.
79. Ali MM, Ghertner R. Broadband access and telemedicine adoption for opioid use disorder treatment in the United States. *J Rural Health.* 2023;39(1):233–239.
80. Weintraub E, Seneviratne C, Anane J, et al. Mobile telemedicine for buprenorphine treatment in rural populations with opioid use disorder. *JAMA Netw Open.* 2021;4(8):e2118487.
81. Uscher-Pines L, Huskamp HA, Mehrotra A. Treating patients with opioid use disorder in their homes: An emerging treatment model. *JAMA.* 2020;324(1):39–40.
82. Massachusetts General Hospital. Kraft Center for Community Health Mobile Addiction Services Toolkit. 2019. https://www.kraftcommunityhealth.org/wp-content/uploads/2020/01/Kraft-Center-Mobile-Addiction-Services-Toolkit.pdf. Accessed Feb. 27, 2023.
83. Landrigan PJ, Rauh VA, Galvez MP. Environmental justice and the health of children. *Mt Sinai J Med.* 2010;77(2):178–187.
84. Office of Disease Prevention and Health Promotion. Healthy People 2030: Neighborhood and built environment. U.S. Department of Health and Human Services. https://health. gov/healthypeople/objectives-and-data/browse-objectives/neighborhood-and-built-environment. 2021. Accessed Feb. 27, 2023.
85. Ellis WR, Dietz WH. A new framework for addressing adverse childhood and community experiences: The building community resilience model. *Acad Pediatr.* 2017;17(7s):S86–S93.
86. Centers for Disease Control and Prevention. Preventing adverse childhood experiences (ACEs): Leveraging the best available evidence. 2019. https://www.cdc.gov/violencepre vention/pdf/preventingACES.pdf. Accessed Feb. 27, 2023.

SOCIAL AND STRUCTURAL DETERMINANTS 135

87. Felitti VJ, Anda RF, Nordenberg D, et al. Relationship of childhood abuse and household dysfunction to many of the leading causes of death in adults: The Adverse Childhood Experiences (ACE) Study. *Am J Prevent Med.* 1998;14(4):245–258.

88. Bethell CD, Carle A, Hudziak J, et al. Methods to assess adverse childhood experiences of children and families: Toward approaches to promote child well-being in policy and practice. *Acad Pediatr.* 2017;17(7s):S51–S69.

89. Merrick MT, Ford DC, Ports KA, et al. Vital signs: Estimated proportion of adult health problems attributable to adverse childhood experiences and implications for prevention – 25 states, 2015-2017. *MMWR Morb Mortal Wkly Rep.* 2019;68(44):999–1005.

90. Office of Disease Prevention and Health Promotion. Health People 2030: Transportation. U.S. Department of Health and Human Services. https://health.gov/healthypeople/obj ectives-and-data/browse-objectives/transportation. 2021. Accessed Feb. 27, 2023.

91. CDC Foundation and Well Being Trust. Thriving together: A springboard for equitable recovery & resilience in communities across America. 2020. https://thriving.us/wp-cont ent/uploads/2020/07/Springboard-Main-Narrative-For-Screen-2.pdf. Accessed Feb. 27, 2023.

92. The Leadership Conference Education Fund. Getting to work: Transportation policy and access to job opportunities. 2011. http://civilrightsdocs.info/pdf/docs/transportat ion/getting-to-work-july20.pdf. Accessed Feb. 27, 2023.

93. Stacy C, Su Y, Noble E, et al. Access to opportunity through equitable transportation: Lessons from four metropolitan regions. 2020. https://www.urban.org/sites/default/ files/publication/102992/access-to-opportunity-through-equitable-transportation_ 0.pdf. Accessed Feb. 27, 2023.

94. Bauerly BC, McCord RF, Hulkower R, Pepin D. Broadband access as a public health issue: The role of law in expanding broadband access and connecting underserved communities for better health outcomes. *J Law Med Ethics.* 2019;47(2 Suppl):39–42.

95. Rafferty AP, Luo H, Egan KL, Bell RA, Gaskins Little NR, Imai S. Rural, suburban, and urban differences in chronic pain and coping among adults in North Carolina: 2018 be-havioral risk factor surveillance system. *Prevent Chronic Dis.* 2021;18:E13.

96. Malenbaum S, Keefe FJ, Williams ACC, Ulrich R, Somers TJ. Pain in its environ-mental context: implications for designing environments to enhance pain control. *Pain.* 2008;134(3):241–244.

97. Forkey HC. Children exposed to abuse and neglect: The effects of trauma on the body and brain. *J Am Acad Matrimonial Lawyers.* 2018;30:307–324.

98. Anderson CE, Broyles ST, Wallace ME, Bazzano LA, Gustat J. Association of the neigh-borhood built environment with incident and prevalent depression in the rural south. *Prevent Chronic Dis.* 2021;18:E67.

99. Helbich M, Hagenauer J, Roberts H. Relative importance of perceived physical and so-cial neighborhood characteristics for depression: A machine learning approach. *Soc Psychiatry Psychiatr Epidemiol.* 2020;55(5):599–610.

100. Pearce M, Garcia L, Abbas A, et al. Association between physical activity and risk of de-pression: A systematic review and meta-analysis. *JAMA Psychiatry.* 2022;79(6):550–559.

101. Hazlehurst MF, Muqueeth S, Wolf KL, Simmons C, Kroshus E, Tandon PS. Park access and mental health among parents and children during the COVID-19 pandemic. *BMC Public Health.* 2022;22(1):800.

102. Nawi AM, Ismail R, Ibrahim F, et al. Risk and protective factors of drug abuse among adolescents: A systematic review. *BMC Public Health.* 2021;21(1):2088.

103. Colpe LJ. Deaths of despair: How connecting opioid data extends the possibilities for su-icide research. 2022. https://www.cdc.gov/surveillance/blogs-stories/deaths-of-dispair. html#print. Accessed Feb. 27, 2023.

104. Sterling P, Platt ML. Why deaths of despair are increasing in the US and not other in-dustrial nations: Insights from neuroscience and anthropology. *JAMA Psychiatry.* 2022;79(4):368–374.

105. Graham C. America's crisis of despair: A federal task force for economic recovery and societal well-being. 2021. https://www.brookings.edu/research/americas-crisis-of-despair-a-federal-task-force-for-economic-recovery-and-societal-well-being/. Accessed Feb. 27, 2023.

106. Rehder K, Lusk J, Chen JI. Deaths of despair: Conceptual and clinical implications. *Cogn Behav Pract.* 2021;28(1):40–52.

107. Tsoi-A-Fatt Bryant R. College preparation for African American students: Gaps in the high school educational experience. 2015. https://www.clasp.org/sites/default/files/public/resources-and-publications/publication-1/College-readiness2-2.pdf. Accessed Feb. 27, 2023.

108. Treuhaft S, Karpyn A. The grocery gap: Who has access to healthy food and why it matters. 2010. https://thefoodtrust.org/wp-content/uploads/2022/06/grocerygap.original.pdf. Accessed Feb. 27, 2023.

109. Johnson-Lawrence V, Scott JB, James SA. Education, perceived discrimination and risk for depression in a southern black cohort. *Aging Ment Health.* 2020;24(11):1872–1878.

110. Legislative Analysis and Public Policy Association. Deflection programs: Summary of state laws. 2021. http://legislativeanalysis.org/wp-content/uploads/2021/07/Deflection-Programs-Summary-of-State-Laws.pdf. Accessed Feb. 27, 2023.

111. Geller A, Fagan J, Tyler T, Link BG. Aggressive policing and the mental health of young urban men. *Am J Public Health.* 2014;104(12):2321–2327.

112. Children's Bureau. Child welfare practice to address racial disproportionality and disparity 2021. https://www.childwelfare.gov/pubpdfs/racial_disproportionality.pdf. Accessed Feb. 27, 2023.

113. Milner J, Kelly D. The need for justice in child welfare. *Child Welfare.* 2021;99.

114. Primack BA, Shensa A, Sidani JE, et al. Social media use and perceived social isolation among young adults in the U.S. *Am J Prevent Med.* 2017;53(1):1–8.

115. Nowland R, Necka EA, Cacioppo JT. Loneliness and social internet use: Pathways to reconnection in a digital world? *Perspect Psychol Sci.* 2018;13(1):70–87.

116. Fernández-Peña R, Molina JL, Valero O. Satisfaction with social support received from social relationships in cases of chronic pain: The influence of personal network characteristics in terms of structure, composition and functional content. *Int J Environ Res Public Health.* 2020;17(8):2706.

117. Verner M, Sirois A, Coutu-Nadeau E, Fournier C, Carriere J, Martel MO. The association between perceived injustice and opioid craving in patients with chronic pain: The mediating role of daily pain intensity, negative affect, and catastrophizing. *J Addict Med.* 2023;17(1):35–41.

118. Sullivan MD, Ballantyne JC. When physical and social pain coexist: Insights into opioid therapy. *Ann Fam Med.* 2021;19(1):79–82.

119. Breedvelt JJF, Tiemeier H, Sharples E, et al. The effects of neighbourhood social cohesion on preventing depression and anxiety among adolescents and young adults: Rapid review. *BJPsych Open.* 2022;8(4):e97.

120. Baranyi G, Sieber S, Cullati S, Pearce JR, Dibben CJL, Courvoisier DS. The longitudinal associations of perceived neighborhood disorder and lack of social cohesion with depression among adults aged 50 years or older: An individual-participant-data meta-analysis from 16 high-income countries. *Am J Epidemiol.* 2020;189(4):343–353.

121. Lê F, Tracy M, Norris FH, Galea S. Displacement, county social cohesion, and depression after a large-scale traumatic event. *Soc Psychiatry Psychiatr Epidemiol.* 2013;48(11):1729–1741.

122. Scott SM, Wallander JL, Cameron L. Protective mechanisms for depression among racial/ethnic minority youth: Empirical findings, issues, and recommendations. *Clin Child Fam Psychol Rev.* 2015;18(4):346–369.

123. National Judicial Opioid Task Force. Convening, collaborating, connecting: Courts as leaders in the crisis of addiction. 2019. http://legislativeanalysis.org/wp-content/uploads/2019/11/Courts-as-Leaders-in-the-Crisis-of-Addiction.pdf. Accessed Feb. 27, 2023.
124. Stanojlović M, Davidson L. Targeting the barriers in the substance use disorder continuum of care with peer recovery support. *Subst Abuse.* 2021;15:1178221820976988.
125. Pettersen H, Landheim A, Skeie I, et al. How social relationships influence substance use disorder recovery: A collaborative narrative study. *Subst Abuse.* 2019;13:1178221819833379.
126. Madras BK, Ahmad NJ, Wen J, Sharfstein J, Prevention T, Recovery Working Group of the Action Collaborative on Countering the U.S. Opioid Epidemic. Improving access to evidence-based medical treatment for opioid use disorder: Strategies to address key barriers within the treatment system. National Academy of Medicine Perspectives. 2020; Discussion Paper.
127. Hirchak KA, Nadeau M, Vasquez A, et al. Centering culture in the treatment of opioid use disorder with American Indian and Alaska Native Communities: Contributions from a National Collaborative Board. *Am J Community Psychol.* 2023 Mar;71(1-2):174–183.
128. Linas BP, Savinkina A, Barbosa C, et al. A clash of epidemics: Impact of the COVID-19 pandemic response on opioid overdose. *J Subst Abuse Treat.* 2021;120:108158.
129. Haley DF, Saitz R. The opioid epidemic during the COVID-19 pandemic. *JAMA.* 2020;324(16):1615–1617.
130. Well Being Trust. Thriving together. https://thriving.us/. 2023. Accessed Mar. 8, 2023.
131. Dawes DE. *The Political Determinants of Health.* Johns Hopkins University Press; 2020.

8

Opioid Taper and Complex Prescription Opioid Dependence

The Role of Depression

Travis I. Lovejoy and Belle Zaccari

8.1 Introduction

Opioid prescribing in the United States reached its peak in 2012, with year-over-year declines observed in the past decade.[1] In addition, higher-risk opioid prescribing—such as prescribing high doses of opioids or co-prescribing of opioids and other controlled substances like benzodiazepines—has steadily declined over this same period.[1,2] These changes have been due, in large part, to programs and policies that assist patients with opioid taper when opioids no longer confer benefit to the patient or when opioid misuse or other high-risk or aberrant behaviors increase the potential for adverse outcomes.[2,3] Unfortunately, some patients do not benefit from opioid tapers. These patients are more likely to have comorbid psychiatric or substance use disorders, are more likely to endorse high pain intensity ratings, and tend to be prescribed opioids at higher doses and for longer periods of time when an opioid taper is initiated.[4]

For many people who live with chronic non-cancer pain, the risks and associated harms of long-term opioid therapy (LTOT) often outweigh its benefits. Data from a randomized controlled trial show that patients with chronic back, hip, or knee osteoarthritis pain experienced no greater improvements in pain severity or functioning over 12 months when prescribed opioid therapy versus non-opioid analgesic medications, while patients prescribed opioids had more medication-related negative side effects.[5] Furthermore, patients in a national retrospective cohort study diagnosed with heterogeneous chronic pain syndromes and prescribed LTOT experienced no

---

Travis I. Lovejoy and Belle Zaccari, *Opioid Taper and Complex Prescription Opioid Dependence* In: *Pain, the Opioid Epidemic, & Depression.* Edited by: Jeffrey F. Scherrer & Jane C. Ballantyne, Oxford University Press.
© Oxford University Press 2024. DOI: 10.1093/9780197675250.003.0008

changes in pain severity, on average, in the year following complete discontinuation of opioids.[6] These data support opioid prescribing guidelines issued by the U.S. Centers for Disease Control and Prevention (CDC) and other health agencies such as the U.S. Department of Veterans Affairs and U.S. Department of Defense that discourage opioid use for chronic non-cancer pain.[7,8] In the current opioid epidemic and concomitant shift to multimodal pain care built on foundations of pain self-management, non-opioid analgesic pharmacotherapy, and non-pharmacologic pain treatment,[9,10] both patients who live with chronic pain and their clinicians face the decision to continue or taper LTOT.

8.2 Defining Opioid Dependence

Opioid dependence has historical connotations as a more severe form of opioid use disorder, based on earlier versions of the *Diagnostic and Statistical Manual of Mental Disorders*[11] and still applied within the International Classification of Diseases (ICD) nosology.[12] A defining characteristic of more severe forms of this disease is *physiologic dependence* on opioids, which manifests as withdrawal symptoms—including opioid cravings, sweating, headaches, muscle aches, loss of appetite, nausea, vomiting, diarrhea, sleep disturbance, anxiety, depression, and agitation. Physiologic dependence on opioids can develop in as little as 2 weeks with regular administration. Sudden cessation of opioids can result in withdrawal symptoms that last anywhere from a few days up to 2 weeks. For patients who have been on LTOT for many years and who subsequently undergo opioid taper, particularly from high doses, these symptoms or some combination of them may last for months.[13] Additional persisting symptoms may include anhedonia and more heightened and intense forms of negative affect, as well as hyperalgesia, which can destabilize patients, disallow a reversal to a normal functional state, and has the potential to lead to drug-seeking behaviors.[14] Ballantyne, Sullivan, and Kolodny termed this phenomenon *complex persistent opioid dependence* (CPOD).[13] Others have termed this phenomenon and its related sequalae *refractory dependence on opioid analgesics*[14] and *opioid induced chronic pain syndrome*.[15] For the purpose of this chapter, we use the term CPOD.

8.3 Pain and Endogenous Opioid Systems

To understand the processes by which individuals may develop CPOD, it is important to consider the contributing factors of their pain experience. Chronic pain is categorized as neuropathic, nociceptive, or nociplastic.[16] Neuropathic pain arises from pathology of the nervous system, most commonly lesions of peripheral nerves. *Physical nociception* describes the central and peripheral nervous system processing of painful stimuli. Nociceptors become activated by stimuli and send signals to the brain to process information about the physical sensation. In the context of harmful stimuli, signals sent to the brain can be helpful in preventing further bodily harm or damage (e.g., pulling one's hand away from a hot stove). *Nociplastic pain* is defined as "pain arising from the altered function of pain-related sensory pathways in the periphery and [central nervous system], causing increased sensitivity."[16] It typically manifests as dull or aching pain, absent tissue, or somatosensory damage and can be localized (e.g., non-structural low back pain) or more diffuse (e.g., fibromyalgia). It is consistent with current ICD definitions of chronic primary pain.[12]

Opioid medications mediate nociceptive neural pathways and can lead to reduced pain sensation. However, they also provide affective relief through reward systems of the brain that involve endogenous opioid systems. Endogenous opioids include enkephalins and endorphins that act as opioid receptor agonists.[17] They are implicated in regulation of metabolism, cardiovascular processes, and may also diminish pain and produce euphoria.[17] Dysregulation of these systems is thought to be a contributing factor of CPOD in some patients. Although opioid medication may be best indicated for acute or nociceptive pain, in practice, opioids have been prescribed for all forms of pain despite clinical guidelines that encourage use of non-opioid analgesic pharmacotherapies and non-pharmacologic pain treatments for patients with chronic pain.[8]

8.4 Opponent Processes

Richard Solomon, a 20th-century psychologist, contended that the primary reaction to an emotional event will be followed by an opposite reaction.[18] For example, something that induces pleasure will be followed by a subsequent feeling of displeasure and vice versa. This phenomenon forms the basis of the *opponent process theory* of drug addiction that describes a state in which chronic drug use produces a desired effect and the organism counters that with an opposing effect to regain a state of homeostasis. In the case of opioids, the medication initially produces analgesia and euphoria, but this is counteracted with hyperalgesia and intense negative affective states, the latter termed *hyperkatifeia*. In hyperkatifeia, negative reward, such as relief of interdose withdrawal symptoms, becomes the driving force for continued opioid use. Over time and continued use, the primary effect of analgesia and euphoria decreases in magnitude and duration, while the counteraction of hyperalgesia and hyperkatifeia intensify and can persist long after opioids are discontinued, as is characteristic of CPOD.[19]

Opponent process theory further contends that the motivation for continued use of a drug is not only to produce the desired primary effect of, in the case of opioids, analgesia and euphoria, but rather to avoid the negative after effects that oppose the primary effects. This negative reinforcement cycle contributes to ongoing use of the substance.

8.5 Allostasis

Allostasis is a process through which an organism achieves stability through change, often in the face of an existing or imminent stressor. The allostatic theory of drug-seeking behavior builds on opponent process theory to explain behavioral manifestations witnessed in CPOD.[20] In a state of homeostasis, the analgesic and euphoric effect of opioids would be precisely counterbalanced by the drug-opposing effect, returning the organism to the pre-drug condition. In this instance, allostatic processes would *not* be activated because the organism naturally returns to its pre-drug state. However, when the drug-opposing effects of hyperalgesia and hyperkatifeia become excessive, allostatic processes activate and increase the organism's desire for the opioid. For patients with CPOD, opioids are no longer effective at reducing pain and reducing negative affect, but continued opioid use for patients with CPOD can lead to an unmanageable allostatic load and chronic pathological states for the patient. As the opponent process strengthens, it eventually dominates, and opioid medication is needed to reduce its pathological effects, including worsening of the original pain.

8.6 Depression in the Context of Opioid Use and Opioid Taper

Depression and pain have been shown to have mutually exacerbating effects, such that increases in pain severity lead to more severe depression, and depressive symptom exacerbation increases reported pain.[21] In addition, patients with chronic pain and a history of depression have a higher likelihood of being prescribed opioid therapy at higher doses and for longer duration compared to patients with chronic pain alone.[22] Some have argued that high rates of LTOT among patients with depression may be a natural self-selection by patients to compensate for reduced endogenous opioid responses to both internal and external stressors that accompany depressive disorders.[23] However, the opponent process theory, described previously, suggests that the person's natural tendency for drug-opposing reactions may counteract the use of prescribed opioids, resulting instead in maintenance or exacerbation of depressive symptom severity instead of relief, as supported by clinical data.[24]

Depression plays a significant role in CPOD as an affective component of the syndrome. Hyperkatifeia is a common feature of an unsuccessful taper,[13] and forcing a taper when patient affect significantly worsens may result in rupture of patient–clinician relationships and other adverse patient outcomes such as suicidality.[25,26] Furthermore, treatment with antidepressant medication has been shown to be associated with successful opioid taper,[27] suggesting that untreated or undertreated depression may be a contributing factor to LTOT maintenance for some patients.

8.7 Treatment in Interdisciplinary Pain Programs During Opioid Taper

For patients with CPOD, extensive support may be required to achieve a successful taper. Frank and colleagues conducted a systematic review of interventions targeting opioid dose reduction and discontinuation to identify intervention characteristics associated with successful patient outcomes.[28] Data from higher-quality studies pointed to interdisciplinary pain programs as the most successful interventions at improving patient-reported pain, function, and quality of life outcomes when undergoing opioid taper. In addition, more intensive treatment (e.g., weekly contact) was also associated with improved outcomes. These programs follow guideline-concordant recommendations of multimodal pain care that will often incorporate pain medicine, nursing, rehabilitation medicine, physical therapy, behavioral pain management, and social work, among other disciplines. Programs offer evidence-based approaches to pain management that include self-management (e.g., heat and cold therapy, transcutaneous electrical nerve stimulation, home exercise programs, pain education, lifestyle changes), psychological and behavioral treatments (e.g., cognitive behavioral therapy, acceptance and commitment therapy for chronic pain), complementary and integrative health approaches (e.g., yoga, Tai Chi, chiropractic care), clinician-guided rehabilitation programs, and interventional pain medicine (e.g., glucocorticoid injections, nerve blocks). Some programs may also include addiction medicine and pharmacy disciplines to oversee management of buprenorphine as an aid for opioid taper.

Because of the high comorbidity of mental health (including depression) symptoms, substance use disorders, and chronic pain, programs will often directly treat or help patients access specialty care that addresses their psychiatric- and substance-related treatment needs. Unfortunately, few programs possess the resources or infrastructure to offer truly collocated, interdisciplinary care in which providers across multiple disciplines work closely as part of a single team. Absent this team-based structure, programs may take the approach of care linkage, in which a care manager helps patients access pain treatment and other needed services across multiple clinics. This is a more common practice in primary care where the majority of opioid tapers are initiated and where structural barriers make interdisciplinary pain, mental health, and substance use disorder treatment more challenging.

8.8 Future Research Directions

Current clinical guidelines and policies discourage opioid use for chronic non-cancer pain.[7,8] In the years subsequent to the original 2016 opioid prescribing guidelines released by the CDC, the authors expressed concern that the guidelines were being misapplied and used as justification to rapidly taper patients off LTOT.[29] These universal tapering policies resulted in a significant reduction of high-risk opioid prescribing[1,2] and have drastically reduced the amount of prescription opioids dispensed in the United States. There continues to be heightened risk of drug overdose at a population level that has not been ameliorated by opioid prescribing policies or practices. In addition, patients on LTOT with low-risk profiles have undergone forced tapers due to systemic and other pressures facing their opioid-prescribing clinicians. Kertesz and Manhapra[26] have suggested that continuing opioid therapy for some patients may be more appropriate than forcing a taper, particularly when patients are of low risk, because forced tapers may create a downward spiral for these patients and ultimately lead to poorer patient outcomes and increased burden to healthcare systems for patients who decompensate. Additional research is needed to better understand those characteristics of patients on LTOT who will benefit from an opioid taper versus those more prone to negative outcomes including severe depression, decreased function, and development of a new or exacerbation of an existing substance use disorder. In addition, further development of clinician training protocols that incorporate principles of patient-centered care and shared decision-making when approaching opioid taper and discontinuation may help preserve trust in the patient–clinician relationship by ensuring patient voices are heard and considered in a collaborative decision-making process.

When patients and clinicians reach a joint decision to undergo an opioid taper, interdisciplinary pain programs could aid in this process, particularly those that incorporate treatment for mental health and substance use disorders. Within primary care, collaborative care models have been shown to improve outcomes of depression,[30] pain, and functioning,[31,32] as well as guideline-concordant opioid prescribing practices.[33] Collaborative care is a team-based care model in which the primary care clinician receives assistance from a care manager around the management of a specific health condition.[34] The care manager is typically a nurse but could involve another discipline (e.g., psychology, social work, pharmacy). A primary goal of collaborative care is to educate patients and improve patients' self-management of the target condition. The care manager, in collaboration with the primary care team, develops treatment plans, taking patient feedback and preferences into consideration; monitors patient outcomes and side effects of treatment; and adjusts treatment as appropriate. Additional activities of the care manager include coordination of specialty care services and navigation of patients through what can sometimes be complex health systems. For patients with CPOD who may require robust interdisciplinary pain and mental health treatment but who may not otherwise have access to this care, collaborative care models administered within the primary care setting may be viable alternatives. Future clinical trials are needed to examine collaborative care specifically for patients with CPOD who have been unsuccessful at tapering LTOT.

Buprenorphine is a partial opioid agonist that is approved by the U.S. Food and Drug Administration (FDA) to treat opioid dependence. It has been proposed as a treatment to aid in opioid taper for patients with CPOD.[35] Yet the field still lacks evidenced-based approaches to opioid taper using buprenorphine for patients with CPOD—including dosing, frequency, and treatment duration—due to the absence of clinical trial data. Until such data are available, clinicians must rely on expert opinion. An example of such guidelines is provided by the U.S. Department of Health and Human Services that address the use of buprenorphine for patients with challenges in tapering opioids.[36,37] In addition, studies that examine implementation of buprenorphine in primary care settings for CPOD are warranted.

8.9 Conclusion

Many patients on LTOT will undergo an opioid taper at some point due to diminished efficacy over time, risk profiles that preclude continued use, or when risks of continued opioid use outweigh benefits. Some patients will experience significant difficulty completing a taper, and initial symptoms of withdrawal may become protracted and accompanied by increased pain and negative affective states. Supporting the whole person and adequately treating pain, depression, and other comorbid conditions utilizing myriad evidence-based approaches has potential to reduce patients' pain and improve functioning and quality of life in the context of opioid taper. Collaborative care models, accompanied by medications for opioid use disorder, such as buprenorphine, may be optimal treatment paradigms for primary care settings where the majority of opioid prescribing happens for chronic pain and where opioid tapers generally initiate, though additional research is needed to further codify treatment protocols and ready these approaches for wider scale implementation.

References

1. Gellad WF, Good CB, Shulkin DJ. Addressing the opioid epidemic in the United States: lessons from the Department of Veterans Affairs. *JAMA Intern Med.* 2017;177(5):611–612.

2. Lin LA, Bohnert AS, Kerns RD, Clay MA, Ganoczy D, Ilgen MA. Impact of the opioid safety initiative on opioid-related prescribing in veterans. *Pain.* 2017;158(5):833–839.
3. Darnall BD, Juurlink D, Kerns RD, et al. International stakeholder community of pain experts and leaders call for an urgent action on forced opioid tapering. *Pain Med.* 2019;20(3):429–433.
4. Davis MP, Digwood G, Mehta Z, McPherson ML. Tapering opioids: A comprehensive qualitative review. *Ann Palliat Med.* 2020;9(2):586–610.
5. Krebs EE, Gravely A, Nugent S, et al. Effect of opioid vs nonopioid medications on pain-related function in patients with chronic back pain or hip or knee osteoarthritis pain: The SPACE randomized clinical trial. *JAMA.* 2018;319(9):872–882.
6. McPherson S, Smith CL, Dobscha SK, et al. Changes in pain intensity after discontinuation of long-term opioid therapy for chronic noncancer pain. *Pain.* 2018;159(10):2097.
7. Card P. VA/DoD clinical practice guideline for opioid therapy for chronic pain. Department of Veterans Affairs, Department of Defense. 2017. https://www.healthquality.va.gov/Guidelines/Pain/Cot/Vadodotcpg022717.Pdf.
8. Dowell D, Ragan KR, Jones CM, Baldwin GT. Centers for Disease Control and Prevention; 2022. CDC Clinical Practice Guideline for Prescribing Opioids for Pain - United States, 2022. [Google Scholar]. https://www.cdc.gov/opioids/patients/guideline.html
9. Becker WC, DeBar LL, Heapy AA, et al. A research agenda for advancing non-pharmacological management of chronic musculoskeletal pain: Findings from a VHA state-of-the-art conference. *J Gen Intern Med.* 2018;33:11–15.
10. Kerns RD, Philip EJ, Lee AW, Rosenberger PH. Implementation of the veterans health administration national pain management strategy. *Translat Behav Med.* 2011;1(4):635–643.
11. Bell CC. DSM-IV: Diagnostic and statistical manual of mental disorders. *JAMA.* 1994;272(10):828–829.
12. Organization WH. *International Statistical Classification of Diseases and related health problems: Alphabetical index.* Vol. 3. World Health Organization; 2004.
13. Ballantyne JC, Sullivan MD, Kolodny A. Opioid dependence vs addiction: A distinction without a difference? *Arch Intern Med.* 2012;172(17):1342–1343.
14. Ballantyne JC, Sullivan MD, Koob GF. Refractory dependence on opioid analgesics. *Pain.* 2019;160(12):2655–2660.
15. Manhapra A. Complex persistent opioid dependence: An opioid-induced chronic pain syndrome. *Curr Treatm Options Oncol.* 2022;23(7):921–935.
16. Fitzcharles M-A, Cohen SP, Clauw DJ, Littlejohn G, Usui C, Häuser W. Nociplastic pain: Towards an understanding of prevalent pain conditions. *Lancet.* 2021;397(10289):2098–2110.
17. Higginbotham JA, Markovic T, Massaly N, Morón JA. Endogenous opioid systems alterations in pain and opioid use disorder. *Front Syst Neurosci.* 2022;16:1014768.
18. Solomon RL, Corbit JD. An opponent-process theory of motivation. *Am Econ Rev.* 1978:12–24.
19. Manhapra A, Arias AJ, Ballantyne JC. The conundrum of opioid tapering in long-term opioid therapy for chronic pain: A commentary. *Subst Abuse.* 2018;39(2):152–161.
20. Ballantyne JC, Koob GF. Allostasis theory in opioid tolerance. *Pain.* 2021;162(9):2315–2319.
21. Kroenke K, Wu J, Bair MJ, Krebs EE, Damush TM, Tu W. Reciprocal relationship between pain and depression: A 12-month longitudinal analysis in primary care. *J Pain.* 2011;12(9):964–973.
22. Braden JB, Sullivan MD, Ray GT, et al. Trends in long-term opioid therapy for noncancer pain among persons with a history of depression. *Gen Hosp Psychiatry.* 2009;31(6):564–570.
23. Sullivan MD. Depression effects on long-term prescription opioid use, abuse, and addiction. *Clin J Pain.* 2018;34(9):878–884.

24. Mazereeuw G, Sullivan MD, Juurlink DN. Depression in chronic pain: Might opioids be responsible? *Pain*. 2018;159(11):2142–2145.
25. Demidenko MI, Dobscha SK, Morasco BJ, Meath TH, Ilgen MA, Lovejoy TI. Suicidal ideation and suicidal self-directed violence following clinician-initiated prescription opioid discontinuation among long-term opioid users. *Gen Hosp Psychiatry*. 2017;47:29–35.
26. Kertesz SG, Manhapra A. The drive to taper opioids: mind the evidence, and the ethics. *Spinal Cord Series Cases*. 2018;4(1):64.
27. Scherrer JF, Salas J, Sullivan MD, et al. Impact of adherence to antidepressants on long-term prescription opioid use cessation. *Br J Psychiatry*. 2018;212(2):103–111.
28. Frank JW, Lovejoy TI, Becker WC, et al. Patient outcomes in dose reduction or discontinuation of long-term opioid therapy: A systematic review. *Ann Intern Med*. 2017;167(3):181–191.
29. Dowell D, Haegerich T, Chou R. No shortcuts to safer opioid prescribing. *N Engl J Med*. 2019;380(24):2285–2287.
30. Gilbody S, Bower P, Fletcher J, Richards D, Sutton AJ. Collaborative care for depression: A cumulative meta-analysis and review of longer-term outcomes. *Arch Intern Med*. 2006;166(21):2314–2321.
31. Dobscha SK, Corson K, Perrin NA, et al. Collaborative care for chronic pain in primary care: A cluster randomized trial. *JAMA*. 2009;301(12):1242–1252.
32. Kroenke K, Bair MJ, Damush TM, et al. Optimized antidepressant therapy and pain self-management in primary care patients with depression and musculoskeletal pain: A randomized controlled trial. *JAMA*. 2009;301(20):2099–2110.
33. Liebschutz JM, Xuan Z, Shanahan CW, et al. Improving adherence to long-term opioid therapy guidelines to reduce opioid misuse in primary care: A cluster-randomized clinical trial. *JAMA Intern Med*. 2017;177(9):1265–1272.
34. Kroenke K, Cheville A. Canons of collaborative care. *J Gen Intern Med*. 2022;37(2):456–458.
35. Manhapra A, Sullivan MD, Ballantyne JC, MacLean RR, Becker WC. Complex persistent opioid dependence with long-term opioids: A gray area that needs definition, better understanding, treatment guidance, and policy changes. *J Gen Intern Med*. 2020;35:964–971.
36. Dowell D, Compton WM, Giroir BP. Patient-centered reduction or discontinuation of long-term opioid analgesics: The HHS guide for clinicians. *JAMA*. 2019;322(19):1855–1856.
37. U.S. Department of Health and Human Services. HHS guide for clinicians on the appropriate dosage reduction or discontinuation of long-term opioid analgesics. 2019. https://www.hhs.gov/system/files/Dosage_Reduction_Discontinuation.pdf.

9

Potential Role for Buprenorphine in the Management of Comorbid Depression Among People with Chronic Pain and Long-Term Opioid Therapy Dependence

Ajay Manhapra, Robert Rosenheck, and William C. Becker

9.1 Introduction

The complex interactions of depression with chronic pain and long-term opioid therapy (LTOT) for chronic pain have been laid out in detail in previous chapters of this volume. It is increasingly recognized that LTOT can be frequently ineffective, and, when it is, opioid taper can also be ineffective.[1-5] Psychiatric instability including worsening depression in addition to worsening pain and disability are shared prominent symptoms in both situations.[1-5] Within this context, buprenorphine has emerged as a preferred choice of LTOT for chronic pain because of its better safety profile and, in cases of ineffective LTOT meriting opioid taper, because of its ability to address the dysphoria of opioid dependence (with and without addiction), the likely key pathological driver in such situations.[1-5] Despite lack of sufficient evidence, buprenorphine is rapidly gaining favor in these scenarios, albeit driven by anecdotal clinical experience and the immediacy and enormity of the need/demand to manage ineffective LTOT safely and effectively.[6,7] The recent U.S. Department of Veterans Affairs (VA) and U.S. Department of Defense (DoD) guidelines on opioid use in chronic pain have endorsed buprenorphine as the first-line choice of opioid if LTOT is being considered.[8] The 2022 guidelines from the U.S. Centers for Disease Control and Prevention (CDC) and the guidelines of the U.S. Department of Health and Human Services (HHS) have both suggested buprenorphine

Ajay Manhapra, Robert Rosenheck, and William C. Becker, *Potential Role for Buprenorphine in the Management of Comorbid Depression Among People with Chronic Pain and Long-Term Opioid Therapy Dependence* In: *Pain, the Opioid Epidemic, & Depression*. Edited by: Jeffrey F. Scherrer & Jane C. Ballantyne, Oxford University Press. © Oxford University Press 2024. DOI: 10.1093/9780197675250.003.0009

as the reasonable option in case of ineffective opioid tapering.[9,10] In addition, the potential of buprenorphine to have antidepressive effects because of its unique pharmacological properties in addition to its actions at the mu opioid receptor (MOR) have been recognized more recently and are being explored in several clinical trials.[11,12] Together, these effects make buprenorphine a potentially useful therapeutic agent when chronic pain, depression, and LTOT dependence co-occur and lead to poor outcomes. In this chapter, we detail the possible ways in which buprenorphine can be utilized in such clinical situations and provide a conceptual framework for exploring buprenorphine utilization among patients with chronic pain and depression on LTOT who are not doing well, and its scientific evaluation.

9.2 History of Therapeutic Use of Buprenorphine to Treat Depression

Medicinal preparations containing opium were used as a panacea or "legitimate" treatment of several diseases including hemorrhage, respiratory illness, malaria, and mood disorders, perhaps because of the ability of opioids to transiently lift the mood and provide relief from distress.[13,14] Opioid-containing products then faded in popularity as the adverse effects of long-term use became evident and medical science progressed to discover newer remedies for diseases that once lacked remedies.[13,14] Since ancient times, the symptoms we commonly associate with major depressive disorder (MDD) (e.g., depressive mood, melancholia, lack of motivation, anxiety, and social withdrawal) have all been recognized as maladies that merit effective treatment, and opioids have been a not infrequent treatment modality.[15] Historic records indicate Sumerians recognized the utility of opium, a dried extract of fluid from the poppy plant (*Papaver somniferum*), in the treatment of depressive symptoms as early as 3400 BC.[15] Assyrians and Egyptians subsequently started the practice of deploying of opium-containing compounds as medicines. On the European front, Homer (8th century BC) described the use of opium-containing medications as a "remedy against grief and grudge," and opium treatment for melancholic maladies were also promoted subsequently by Hippocrates (400 BC) and Galen (200 AD).[15] In the rich medieval Arabic culture, Avicenna (980–1037 AD) described the utility of opium in treating depression symptoms.[15]

Opium, mixed with alcohol, was reportedly introduced into the European pharmacopeia as laudanum in the 1500s, and the use of opium-containing products for treatment of depression symptoms in Europe expanded steadily over the next few centuries.[15] Opium was an integral pharmacological intervention used during the growth of the German "Romantic Psychiatry" movement in the 1600s and 1700s, the conceptual predecessor of the modern psychiatric treatment paradigms.[15] "Opiumkur," roughly translated from German to English as "Opium cure" (escalating doses of tincture of opium given daily and then weaned off over 2 months), was established as an effective cure for treatment-refractory depression (TRD) delivered through asylum-based treatment programs in the late 18th and 19th centuries largely due to the work of German psychiatrists.[15,16] This practice seems to have percolated from specialists treating severe psychiatric disorders in the controlled environments of asylums to general practitioners in communities using opium products extensively in the treatment of less severe depression symptoms like insomnia, "hysteria," and anxiety.[15] Descriptions of the benefit of opium in depressive symptoms and characterization of opium as the "happiness" drug started appearing in European literature like the popular book *Confessions of an English Opium-Eater* (1821) by Thomas de Quincey.[16] As the use of opium became popular, clinicians also started recognizing that dependence on opium could create depressive symptoms on its own, coining the term "morphinism."[15] Despite the growing burden and awareness of opioid addiction and subsequent restrictive laws, various opioid regimens continued to be widely used in treatment of TRD in Europe as recently as the years immediately after World War II.

Use of opioids in depression ebbed considerably after the introduction of monoaminergic medications as effective treatment during 1950s and 1960s.[16] However, the discovery of the endorphin system and opiate receptors reawakened interest in opioids as a treatment option in depression in the 1970s. It was hypothesized that a defectively operating endogenous endorphin system might have a pathogenic role in endogenous depression and that stimulation of the endorphin system would provide an avenue for depression treatment. Results of early clinical trials treating depression based on this "deficient endorphin system" model suggested that beta-endorphin infusion may be beneficial in alleviating depression.[17-19] Merging the prior experience with "opium cure" in TRD and the newer realization that opioids act through the stimulation of opioid receptors and the endogenous endorphin system, buprenorphine was trialed as the prototypical opioid for depression treatment in the late 1970s and early 1980s.[20,21] Buprenorphine was appealing because of its ability to easily penetrate the blood–brain barrier, relatively low dependence risk, and quick onset of action.[12,20,21] The first double-blind crossover study in 1982, by Emrich et al. (placebo followed by buprenorphine and then placebo, all blinded), reported a mean 40% reduction in Hamilton Rating Scale for Depression (HAM-D) scores with low dose (0.2 mg) sublingual buprenorphine among 50% of patients with TRD who had failed conventional treatments.[20] This was followed by a series of small studies over the next two decades showing continued benefits of treatment of TRD with low-dose buprenorphine.[21,22] As sublingual buprenorphine combined with naltrexone emerged as a first-line treatment of opioid use disorder in the United States after 2003, several studies reported improved outcomes among those with comorbid depression and opioid use disorder (OUD) compared to those with OUD and no depression.[22]

With the growing knowledge of opioid receptor biology over the past several decades, kappa opioid receptor (KOR) antagonism was identified as a unique characteristic of buprenorphine compared to other opioids used as therapeutic agents, this in addition to its agonist action on the MOR shared with other opioids.[12,22,23] The MOR is the main therapeutic target of opioids, and MOR stimulation is thought to account for the main opioid effects including euphoria, sedation, analgesia, reward, and dysphoria.[12,22,23] On the other hand, KOR antagonism was found to be associated with an antidysphoric effect, which has utility in treatment of depression.[12,22,23] Subsequently, a combination of buprenorphine with the MOR antagonist samidorphan to ameliorate undesirable effects like misuse and OUD mediated by the MOR and isolating the KOR actions of buprenorphine has been studied as depression treatment in several clinical trials with promising results.[12,22-24] There are also reports that people with co-occurring chronic pain and depression appear to benefit more from buprenorphine compared to other opioids, with buprenorphine also associated with lower rates of misuse and suicidal intent.[25,26] Interest and knowledge regarding the utility of buprenorphine as a therapeutic agent in depression with or without chronic pain or OUD has grown substantially. We provide a brief review of the available data regarding the use of buprenorphine to treat depression in Sections 4–6 of this chapter.

9.3 Buprenorphine Basic Pharmacology

The effects of opioids pertinent to analgesia, euphoria, and antidepressive properties are achieved through their binding and activation of the MOR, KOR, and delta opioid receptors (DOR) as well as the nociceptin/orphanin FQ (NOP) receptors in the endogenous opioid system of the brain.[12,27–29] The balance between MOR and KOR agonist and antagonistic actions is considered a major factor in maintaining functionally adaptive mood states.[12,27–29] In addition to its analgesic effect, MOR stimulation results in several other effects pertinent to mechanisms of major depressive disorder (MDD). Agonism of MOR mediates the processing of natural rewards and reward-associated reinforcing properties of opioid and non-opioid drugs.[12,27–29] MOR activation is also critical in driving motivation for participating in socially rewarding activities. Impaired reward processing is considered a major mechanism driving MDD and also the connecting pathophysiological link between depression and pain.[30] Impairment of socially hedonic behaviors is also a significant clinical element of depressive disorders.[27] Depressive disorders are associated with a downregulation of the MOR receptors [12,27–29] However, MOR activation is also associated with the development of addictive behaviors.[12,27–29]

Dissimilar to the MOR receptor system, the KOR receptor system has been characterized as the "anti-reward" system.[27] KOR activation is associated with anhedonia, depression, low motivation, and stress-associated aversive moods, all critical elements of depressive disorder.[12,27–29] KOR system dysregulation is considered an important element of clinical depressive states.[12,27–29] Consistent with this, KOR antagonists have been associated with antidepressant effects in experimental and clinical studies.[12,27–29]

In addition to MOR agonism, buprenorphine also has a potent KOR antagonist action. This combination of MOR agonism and KOR antagonism makes buprenorphine a uniquely compelling therapeutic agent in the treatment of depression, especially in the context of co-existing pain and opioid dependence.[12,27–29]

While the oral absorption of buprenorphine is poor because of first-pass metabolism, it is efficiently absorbed through oral mucosa with high bioavailability.[31] This makes sublingual and buccal administration effective in therapeutic use.[31] Limited absorption through the transdermal route has been overcome effectively by newer transdermal formulations. Because of high receptor affinity and low receptor dissociation, buprenorphine has a long half-life compared to other opioids.[31] It is also a highly potent analgesic with reduced adverse effects like respiratory depression (due to ceiling effect) compared to other opioids, thus making it relatively safer than many other analgesics.[31] The unique combination of long duration of action, high receptor affinity, effective MOR agonism, and low side effects led to the establishment of buprenorphine as a favored option for the treatment of the negative consequences of opioid dependence in OUD and opioid addiction.[32]

9.4 Low-Dose Buprenorphine in Treatment-Refractory Depression Among Opioid-Naïve Individuals

Although the current appeal of buprenorphine for management of TRD is largely focused on its unique KOR antagonist effect, its experimental use started in the 1970s, based on the hypothesis that it would be a better agonist of the newly discovered endorphin system because of its high blood–brain barrier penetration and low side effects.[12,20,21] The rapid onset of action of opioids, including buprenorphine, when compared to other antidepressants was felt to offer a definite clinical advantage.[22,23] As described above, the first double-blind crossover study in 1982, by Emrich et al., reported substantial clinically meaningful relief from depression with low-dose (0.2 mg) sublingual buprenorphine among 50% of patients with TRD unresponsive to conventional treatments,[20] with similar results observed in several follow-up studies with low-dose buprenorphine, albeit with small numbers of enrolled patients and open-label designs.[20–22,33] However, in a small randomized control trial (RCT) with limited data reported, augmentation of standard depression treatment with low-dose (0.4 mg) buprenorphine was not found to be superior to placebo.[22,34] Several other RCTs that followed also did not show significant benefit individually.[24]

As the specific roles of KOR in depression and MOR in addictive behaviors became more recognized, extracting the beneficial KOR antagonist effect of buprenorphine without adverse MOR effects became more appealing in the treatment of TRD. In the first of the RCTs evaluating the benefit of 1:1 combination (4 mg and 4 mg) of buprenorphine and samidorphan, a selective MOR antagonist in TRD, Ehrich et al. found only marginal benefit compared to placebo.[35] Several larger RCTs that followed also showed marginal benefits for the buprenorphine–samidorphan combination.[24] In a systematic review of 11 RCTs evaluating buprenorphine or buprenorphine–samidorphan combination against placebos in TRD with data on a total of 1,699 patients, buprenorphine resulted in a small, clinically meaningful reduction in depressive symptoms.[24] Buprenorphine was well tolerated and had no significant abuse liability or dependency in studies that lasted up to only 8 weeks.[24] Longer-term follow-up data are needed regarding benefits, safety, abuse liability, and dependency risks in the use of buprenorphine for TRD among opioid-naïve individuals.

9.5 Buprenorphine in Treatment of Depression Comorbid with Opioid Use Disorder

People with OUD have a significantly higher prevalence of depression (up to 50% or more) compared to the general population. Depression in OUD is associated with poor treatment compliance, higher prevalence of other drug use and drug use disorders, and lower rates of long-term remission. In cases of TRD among opioid-naïve individuals, low-dose buprenorphine is used to stimulate or manipulate the inadequately functioning endogenous endorphin system, unexposed previously to regular exogenous opioid use, with a primary goal of decreasing depression. On the other hand, in OUD, high-dose buprenorphine is used to modify the endogenous opioid system that is malfunctioning due to the dependence on other exogenous opioids. Thus, in buprenorphine treatment of OUD, improvements in depressive symptoms are likely secondary to gains from primary treatment of opioid dependence.

In a small, open-label study among people with OUD by Kosten et al. published in 1990, nearly two-thirds of participants with depression and OUD (19 patients) showed significant improvement in depression with buprenorphine (2–8 mg) when used for treatment of OUD, with the onset of benefit occurring within the first 2 weeks among more than 80% of patients.[36] A similar more recent study also showed similar benefit with regards to depression with buprenorphine treatment for both heroin abuse and prescription OUD.[37] The improvement was more marked among those with prescription OUD.[37] Improved depression symptoms among those with comorbid depression and OUD was reported from several RCTs testing the effectiveness of higher doses of buprenorphine (8–32 mg) in the treatment of OUD.[22] These results suggest that buprenorphine is associated with antidepressant effects at a wide range of doses, and these benefits tend to materialize quickly compared to other conventional antidepressant therapies.[22] There is some suggestion that buprenorphine treatment for OUD may be superior to methadone treatment in controlling comorbid depressive symptoms, but the data are limited and inconclusive.[22,38–40]

Readers are referred to Namchuk et al.[22] for a more detailed clinically pertinent review of the benefits of buprenorphine treatment in TRD among opioid-naïve individuals and among those with comorbid depression and OUD.

9.6 Buprenorphine in Treatment of Depression Comorbid with Chronic Pain and Long-Term Opioid Therapy

Literature regarding the use of buprenorphine for treatment of depression associated with LTOT for chronic pain is scant. However, as laid out in previous chapters, the prevalence of depression is high among people with chronic pain, especially high-impact chronic pain, and comorbid depression is associated with poor pain control and treatment outcomes related to both depression and chronic pain.[41–45] Depression is associated with increased odds of receiving prescription opioids and greater risk for opioid misuse among people with chronic pain, often regardless of pain severity.[46–49] Although it is generally advised that LTOT should be avoided among people with comorbid psychiatric disorders, patients with both chronic pain and comorbid psychiatric disorders such as depression are more likely to receive LTOT in general, at higher doses, and to experience more adverse effects of LTOT, including addiction, overdose, and suicide, reflecting the so-called adverse selection of patients for LTOT.[46,50] LTOT is also associated with development of TRD among people with chronic pain and preexisting depression.[51] Conversely, among people without a recent history of depression, LTOT is associated with an increased incidence of depression, more so with longer duration and higher doses of LTOT regardless of the type of opioids.[52–56] New-onset depression following LTOT also appears to be more severe than depression that onsets in patients with chronic pain who are not on opioids.[57] Opioid tapering, the U.S. Centers for Disease Control and Prevention's recommended management strategy for when harms outweigh benefits of LTOT, is also associated with increased psychiatric destabilization, overdose, and suicide, in addition to worsening pain that can last long after LTOT tapering or discontinuation.

Thus, the relationship between LTOT and depression among people with chronic pain appears to be complex and bidirectional. Although opioid therapy can provide short-term relief from depression for some, LTOT is associated with worsening depression among many with preexisting depression and incident depression among those without prior depression.[5] Paradoxically, worsening or new depression and suicidality can emerge with opioid tapering and persist for months and even years.[5] This LTOT-associated depression is often refractory to conventional depression treatments.[5] We and others have proposed that development, worsening, and treatment refractoriness of depression and other psychiatric disorders along with pain associated with LTOT initiation, continuation, and tapering, are part of the clinical phenomenology of an *opioid-induced chronic pain syndrome* (OICP).[5] We describe OICP as a highly prevalent maladaptive form of opioid dependence associated with LTOT, or a complex persistent opioid dependence (CPOD) state, that is distinct from OUD when loss of control of opioid use predominates.[5] The new onset and worsening of depression and its treatment refractoriness associated with LTOT initiation, continuation, and deprescribing are viewed as a symptom of OICP rather than as a separate clinical entity of major depressive disorder.[5] Based on this conceptualization and borrowing principles from OUD treatment, use of long-acting opioids like buprenorphine to treat CPOD, explicitly without an expectation of analgesia, combined with behavioral modifications has been proposed as an effective treatment of TRD, psychiatric destabilization, pain, and debility (aka OICP) associated with LTOT continuation and tapering.[5] In such clinical destabilization due to LTOT, a switch from LTOT agents to buprenorphine with a shift in focus from the goal of analgesia, which often was not achieved on LTOT anyway, to treatment of CPOD can be expected to stabilize and improve concurrent psychiatric disorders including depression, pain, and debility of the individual without much simultaneous improvement in pain, but this clinical improvement may later translate to a better functional life with or without pain.[1,5] Consistent with the above notion, a recent qualitative study of people on LTOT who were switched to buprenorphine from other LTOT agents reported that they experienced functional improvement and improved overall psychological well-being without much decrease in pain.[7] In the subsequent sections, we provide a brief description of CPOD with the clinical phenomenology of OICP and our approach to buprenorphine-based treatment.

9.7 How Long-Term Opioid Use for Pain Can Lead to More Pain and Depression

People with chronic pain also experience several additional symptoms including depression, anxiety, social avoidance, fatigue, and insomnia, all of which are key features of depression.[5,58] Although often conceptualized as separate clinical entities with causal connections (e.g. "pain leads to depression"), these non-pain symptoms are experienced concurrently with pain.[58,59] In addition, chronic pain exacerbations are often dominated by exacerbations of non-pain experiences and debility without an increase in pain.[60,61] Thus, what people report as "pain" is often dominated by several symptoms or experiences other than pain, including depression. In the same vein, pain relief is not merely a reduction in pain mediated by the nociceptive system but a complex experience involving relief from distress due to several other experiences like depression, anxiety, and insomnia.[1,62–66] Non-pain symptoms like depression and anxiety also appear to drive opioid use and misuse among people on LTOT for chronic pain more than pain does.[49,59,67,68] Pain relief from opioid use is also a global relief from multiple distressing symptoms, including depression, mediated by its effect on the reward system and not just mere analgesia achieved through anti-nociceptive mechanisms.[1,62–66] In addition, opioid use also enhances the placebo effect and internal motivation for social functioning.[69–72] Thus, when effective—which tends to be only in the beginning of treatment—opioids function as distress relief medications that enhance placebo effects and may allow improved functioning, not as merely analgesics.[1,5,73]

Because relief is coded as a highly valued reward by the brain, mediated through a system that drives automatized learning of rewarding behaviors, the brain undergoes several adaptations with repeated use of opioids that modify the polysymptomatic pain experience.[1,5,73]

A prominent adaptation is the development of a counterbalancing opponent effect to global relief: a pain that is experienced concurrently with relief and persists after the relief effect wears off as rebound/withdrawal pain.[2,4,74–76] A broader physiological adaptation called *allostasis* also emerges in combination with this growing opponent effect, termed together as the "allostatic opponent effect," which resets the baseline pain and polysymptomatic psychological distress experience to higher set points around which the pain-distress/relief cycles fluctuate.[4,66,73–77] Disability and suffering that includes anxiety, anger, irritability, depression, concentration problems, sleep problems, fatigue, and lethargy can also similarly increase as a part of the increasing allostatic opponent effect.[1,4,66] This overall clinical worsening associated with allostatic opponent effect may persist or worsen whether LTOT is continued, increased, or decreased.[5] This clinical decline associated with allostatic opponent adaptations may persist and even worsen for months or years after LTOT cessation or dose decrease. This persistence of pain and psychological distress is commonly referred to as *protracted withdrawal/ abstinence syndrome*.[1,3,5,78,79] Worsening anhedonia and depression is often a key component of protracted abstinence syndrome, too.[1,3,5,73,78,79] The allostatic opponent adaptations are considered the driving neurobehavioral mechanisms involved in the development of opioid tolerance and dependence.[4] Thus, maladaptive opioid dependence (aka OICP) offers a valid explanation for high rates of incident depression and worsening of preexisting depression and their treatment refractoriness with LTOT initiation, continuation, and deprescribing.[1,5,73] This conceptualization also provides the framework for the use of buprenorphine and behavioral modifications in the treatment of OICP and associated depression.[1,5,73]

9.8 Buprenorphine Use in LTOT Dependence-Induced OICP and Associated Depression

Because there are limited RCT data on the use of buprenorphine to treat LTOT dependence-induced OICP and associated depression, the urgency of the opioid crisis has pushed the widespread uptake of pragmatic clinical practice. Here, we provide a summary of our clinical approach—one which may be useful to clinicians and researchers.

First, it is critical not to confuse using buprenorphine as LTOT for chronic pain among patients who are opioid-naïve and buprenorphine treatment for both OICP and depression due to LTOT. In the first scenario, in buprenorphine use for LTOT in chronic pain, the endogenous system previously unexposed to long-term use of exogenous opioids is stimulated and modified with long-term use of low-dose transdermal and buccal formulations of buprenorphine to improve function and pain control. In the second scenario, in the treatment of OICP and related depression, high-dose buprenorphine is used to modify the endogenous opioid system rendered dysfunctional from the use of long-term exogenous opioids and improve overall function, which in turn might lead to better control of pain and depression. Among people with LTOT-induced depression and OICP, allostatic adaptations of endogenous opioid systems in response to long-term opioid use with a specific dose, pattern, and effect expectancy creates a physiological stability associated with poor function and worsened pain and depression. Buprenorphine-based treatment in such situations is conceptualized as a different dose, with the pattern of use of a longer-acting opioid with different expectations and behavioral modifications to achieve a physiological stability associated with better function and improved pain control and depression. For example, consider the case of a patient who developed worsening pain, depression, and function on sustained-action morphine 100 mg twice a day and immediate-release oxycodone 5 mg every 6 hours as needed for breakthrough pain. This patient was started on opioid taper for LTOT ineffectiveness and unacceptable level of opioid risk, and this led to further worsening of pain and other symptoms including depression. Buprenorphine/naloxone 8 mg/2 mg twice a day sublingually without as-needed use of short-acting opioids was introduced as treatment in this case. Here, high-dose, longer-acting buprenorphine is expected to achieve a sufficiently higher sustained occupancy of opioid receptors compared to the waxing and waning low-level receptor occupancy pattern observed with the previous regimen. Such a sustained high level of receptor occupancy may provide greater physiological stability that then may be associated with improved function and mood and not necessarily lesser pain. A similar response was recently reported by a qualitative study of patients on LTOT transitioned to buprenorphine.[7] It is important to set up the treatment expectations appropriately. The patient should understand and accept that buprenorphine is used here as a treatment of maladaptive opioid dependence and not as an alternate analgesic agent, as in the practice of opioid analgesic rotation, and that the goal of treatment is improvement of overall function, mood, sleep, etc., not necessarily reducing pain. Patients with OICP typically have poor pain control so messaging around "feeling better overall/ feeling less weighed down" may resonate and may encourage patients to think more broadly about their global symptom experience. Patients on ineffective LTOT often have waxing and waning of pain and mood symptoms with a learned practice of managing these momentary swings pharmacologically. Instead, the patient should be advised to manage these expected transient escalations in pain and mood using behavioral techniques. The patient should take advantage of the early mood and functional improvements experienced with a switch to buprenorphine to work with providers to improve even further. The long-term goal should be to achieve and maintain a life with improved function and psychiatric stability on buprenorphine with the patient subsequently training themselves to maintain the functional level with lower and lower doses of buprenorphine and eventually without any opioids. Although this approach is intuitively appealing and a growing body of observational studies support it, more RCTs are required to validate it.

9.9 Conclusion

With more than 7 million people likely to have been tapered off LTOT since 2014 and more than 7 million still on LTOT in the United States—with many reporting poor health and functioning—it is likely that emerging or worsening depression as a consequence of LTOT is a major but poorly recognized problem among people with chronic pain.[54,55,57,80] Buprenorphine treatment of opioid dependence offers an intriguing opportunity to manage these patients who are commonly refractory to depression treatments. It is not clear whether KOR antagonism unique to buprenorphine adds further benefits. More focused research is required to characterize the phenomenology of depression emerging or worsening with LTOT and its deprescribing. The utility of buprenorphine in treating such LTOT-induced depression needs further examination.

References

1. Manhapra A, Arias AJ, Ballantyne JC. The conundrum of opioid tapering in long-term opioid therapy for chronic pain: A commentary. *Subst Abuse.* 2018;39(2):152–161.
2. Ballantyne JC, Sullivan MD, Koob GF. Refractory dependence on opioid analgesics. *Pain.* 2019;160(12):2655–2660.
3. Manhapra A, Sullivan MD, Ballantyne JC, MacLean RR, Becker WC. Complex persistent opioid dependence with long-term opioids: A gray area that needs definition, better understanding, treatment guidance, and policy changes. *J Gen Intern Med.* 2020;35(Suppl 3):964–971.
4. Ballantyne JC, Koob GF. Allostasis theory in opioid tolerance. *Pain.* 2021; 162(9):2315–2319.
5. Manhapra A. Complex persistent opioid dependence: An opioid-induced chronic pain syndrome. *Curr Treat Options Oncol.* 2022;23(7):921–935.
6. Oldfield BJ, Edens EL, Agnoli A, et al. Multimodal treatment options, including rotating to buprenorphine, within a multidisciplinary pain clinic for patients on risky opioid

regimens: A quality improvement study. *Pain Med (Malden, Mass)*. 2018;19(suppl_1):S38–S45.

7. Edmond SN, Wesolowicz DM, Snow JL, et al. Qualitative analysis of patient perspectives of buprenorphine after transitioning from long-term, full-agonist opioid therapy among veterans with chronic pain. *J Pain*. 2024 Jan;25(1):132–141.

8. Department of Veterans Affairs/Department of Defense. Clinical practice guideline for the use of opioids in the management of chronic pain. Use of opioids in the management of chronic pain. 2022. https://www.healthquality.va.gov/guidelines/Pain/cot/VADoDOpioidsCPG.pdf. Accessed Oct. 3, 2023.

9. Dowell D, Ragan KR, Jones CM, Baldwin GT, Chou R. CDC clinical practice guideline for prescribing opioids for pain: United States, 2022. *MMWR Recomm Rep*. 2022;71(3):1–95.

10. Dowell D, Compton WM, Giroir BP. Patient-centered reduction or discontinuation of long-term opioid analgesics: The HHS guide for clinicians. *JAMA*. 2019:1–3.

11. Stefanowski B, Antosik-Wojcinska A, Swiecicki L. The use of buprenorphine in the treatment of drug-resistant depression: An overview of the studies. *Psychiatr Pol*. 2020;54(2):199–207.

12. Pecina M, Karp JF, Mathew S, Todtenkopf MS, Ehrich EW, Zubieta JK. Endogenous opioid system dysregulation in depression: Implications for new therapeutic approaches. *Molecular psychiatry*. 2019;24(4):576–587.

13. Lomax E. The uses and abuses of opiates in nineteenth-century England. *Bull Hist Med*. 1973;47(2):167–176.

14. Berridge V. Victorian opium eating: Response to opiate use in nineteenth century England. *Vic Stud*. 1978;21(4):437–461.

15. Weber MM, Emrich HM. Current and historical concepts of opiate treatment in psychiatric disorders. *Int Clin Psychopharmacol*. 1988;3(3):255–266.

16. Tenore PL. Psychotherapeutic benefits of opioid agonist therapy. *J Addict Dis*. 2008;27(3):49–65.

17. Gerner RH, Catlin DH, Gorelick DA, Hui KK, Li CH. Beta-endorphin: Intravenous infusion causes behavioral change in psychiatric inpatients. *Arch Gen Psychiatry*. 1980;37(6):642–647.

18. Kline NS, Li CH, Lehmann HE, Lajtha A, Laski E, Cooper T. Beta-endorphin-induced changes in schizophrenic and depressed patients. *Arch Gen Psychiatry*. 1977;34(9):1111–1113.

19. Pickar D, Davis GC, Schulz SC, et al. Behavioral and biological effects of acute beta-endorphin injection in schizophrenic and depressed patients. *Am J Psychiatry*. 1981;138(2):160–166.

20. Emrich HM, Vogt P, Herz A. Possible antidepressive effects of opioids: Action of buprenorphine. *Ann NY Acad Sci*. 1982;398:108–112.

21. Emrich HM, Vogt P, Herz A, Kissling W. Antidepressant effects of buprenorphine. *Lancet*. 1982;2(8300):709.

22. Namchuk AB, Lucki I, Browne CA. Buprenorphine as a treatment for major depression and opioid use disorder. *Adv Drug Alcohol Res*. 2022;2:10254.

23. Browne CA, Jacobson ML, Lucki I. Novel targets to treat depression: Opioid-based therapeutics. *Harv Rev Psychiatry*. 2020;28(1):40–59.

24. Riblet NB, Young-Xu Y, Shiner B, Schnurr PP, Watts BV. The efficacy and safety of buprenorphine for the treatment of depression: A systematic review and meta-analysis. *J Psychiatric Res*. 2023;161:393–401.

25. Scherrer JF, Salas J, Grucza R, et al. Depression and buprenorphine treatment in patients with non-cancer pain and prescription opioid dependence without comorbid substance use disorders. *J Affect Disord*. 2021;278:563–569.

26. Coplan PM, Sessler NE, Harikrishnan V, Singh R, Perkel C. Comparison of abuse, suspected suicidal intent, and fatalities related to the 7-day buprenorphine transdermal

patch versus other opioid analgesics in the National Poison Data System. *Postgrad Med.* 2017;129(1):55–61.

27. Jelen LA, Stone JM, Young AH, Mehta MA. The opioid system in depression. *Neurosci Biobehav Rev.* 2022;140:104800.

28. Browne CA, Lucki I. Targeting opioid dysregulation in depression for the development of novel therapeutics. *Pharmacol Ther.* 2019;201:51–76.

29. Berrocoso E, Sanchez-Blazquez P, Garzon J, Mico JA. Opiates as antidepressants. *Curr Pharmaceut Design.* 2009;15(14):1612–1622.

30. Rizvi SJ, Gandhi W, Salomons T. Reward processing as a common diathesis for chronic pain and depression. *Neurosci Biobehav Rev.* 2021;127:749–760.

31. Gudin J, Fudin J. A narrative pharmacological review of buprenorphine: A unique opioid for the treatment of chronic pain. *Pain Ther.* 2020;9(1):41–54.

32. Heidbreder C, Fudala PJ, Greenwald MK. History of the discovery, development, and FDA-approval of buprenorphine medications for the treatment of opioid use disorder. *Drug Alcohol Depend Rep.* 2023;6:100133.

33. Karp JF, Butters MA, Begley AE, et al. Safety, tolerability, and clinical effect of low-dose buprenorphine for treatment-resistant depression in midlife and older adults. *J Clin Psychiatry.* 2014;75(8):e785–793.

34. Lin C, Karim HT, Pecina M, et al. Low-dose augmentation with buprenorphine increases emotional reactivity but not reward activity in treatment resistant mid- and late-life depression. *Neuroimage Clin.* 2019;21:101679.

35. Ehrich E, Turncliff R, Du Y, et al. Evaluation of opioid modulation in major depressive disorder. *Neuropsychopharmacology.* 2015;40(6):1448–1455.

36. Kosten TR, Morgan C, Kosten TA. Depressive symptoms during buprenorphine treatment of opioid abusers. *J Subst Abuse Treatm.* 1990;7(1):51–54.

37. Romero-Gonzalez M, Shahanaghi A, DiGirolamo GJ, Gonzalez G. Buprenorphine-naloxone treatment responses differ between young adults with heroin and prescription opioid use disorders. *Am J Addict.* 2017;26(8):838–844.

38. Dean AJ, Bell J, Christie MJ, Mattick RP. Depressive symptoms during buprenorphine vs. methadone maintenance: Findings from a randomised, controlled trial in opioid dependence. *Eur Psychiatry.* 2004;19(8):510–513.

39. Maremmani I, Pani PP, Pacini M, Perugi G. Substance use and quality of life over 12 months among buprenorphine maintenance-treated and methadone maintenance-treated heroin-addicted patients. *J Subst Abuse Treatm.* 2007;33(1):91–98.

40. Gerra G, Borella F, Zaimovic A, et al. Buprenorphine versus methadone for opioid dependence: Predictor variables for treatment outcome. *Drug Alcohol Depend.* 2004;75(1):37–45.

41. IsHak WW, Wen RY, Naghdechi L, et al. Pain and depression: A systematic review. *Harv Rev Psychiatry.* 2018;26(6):352–363.

42. Israel JA. The impact of residual symptoms in major depression. *Pharmaceuticals (Basel).* 2010;3(8):2426–2440.

43. Goesling J, Lin LA, Clauw DJ. Psychiatry and pain management: At the intersection of chronic pain and mental health. *Curr Psychiatry Rep.* 2018;20(2):12.

44. Hooten WM. Chronic pain and mental health disorders: Shared neural mechanisms, epidemiology, and treatment. *Mayo Clin Proc.* 2016;91(7):955–970.

45. Workman EA, Hubbard JR, Felker BL. Comorbid psychiatric disorders and predictors of pain management program success in patients with chronic pain. *Prim Care Companion J Clin Psychiatry.* 2002;4(4):137–140.

46. Sullivan MD. Depression effects on long-term prescription opioid use, abuse, and addiction. *Clin J Pain.* 2018;34(9):878–884.

47. Jaiswal A, Scherrer JF, Salas J, van den Berk-Clark C, Fernando S, Herndon CM. Differences in the association between depression and opioid misuse in chronic low back pain versus chronic pain at other locations. *Healthcare (Basel).* 2016;4(2):34.

BUPRENORPHINE 163

48. Rubenstein W, Grace T, Croci R, Ward D. The interaction of depression and prior opioid use on pain and opioid requirements after total joint arthroplasty. *Arthroplast Today.* 2018;4(4):464–469.
49. Goesling J, Henry MJ, Moser SE, et al. Symptoms of depression are associated with opioid use regardless of pain severity and physical functioning among treatment-seeking patients with chronic pain. *J Pain.* 2015;16(9):844–851.
50. Howe CQ, Sullivan MD. The missing 'p' in pain management: How the current opioid epidemic highlights the need for psychiatric services in chronic pain care. *Gen Hosp Psychiatry.* 2014;36(1):99–104.
51. Scherrer JF, Salas J, Sullivan MD, et al. The influence of prescription opioid use duration and dose on development of treatment resistant depression. *Prevent Med.* 2016;91:110–116.
52. Scherrer JF, Salas J, Lustman PJ, Burge S, Schneider FD. Change in opioid dose and change in depression in a longitudinal primary care patient cohort. *Pain.* 2015;156(2):348–355.
53. Scherrer JF, Svrakic DM, Freedland KE, et al. Prescription opioid analgesics increase the risk of depression. *J Gen Intern Med.* 2014;29(3):491–499.
54. Scherrer JF, Salas J, Bucholz KK, et al. New depression diagnosis following prescription of codeine, hydrocodone or oxycodone. *Pharmacoepidemiol Drug Saf.* 2016;25(5):560–568.
55. Scherrer JF, Salas J, Copeland LA, et al. Prescription opioid duration, dose, and increased risk of depression in 3 large patient populations. *Ann Fam Med.* 2016;14(1):54–62.
56. Scherrer JF, Salas J, Miller-Matero LR, et al. Long-term prescription opioid users' risk for new-onset depression increases with frequency of use. *Pain.* 2022;163(8):1581–1589.
57. Scherrer JF, Salas J, Schneider FD, et al. Characteristics of new depression diagnoses in patients with and without prior chronic opioid use. *J Affect Disord.* 2017;210:125–129.
58. Manhapra A. Rethinking clinically significant pain: A marker of recovery rather than a warning of injury. *Pain.* 2023;164(3):e174.
59. Gilam G, Sturgeon JA, You DS, Wasan AD, Darnall BD, Mackey SC. Negative affect-related factors have the strongest association with prescription opioid misuse in a cross-sectional cohort of patients with chronic pain. *Pain Med (Malden, Mass).* 2020;21(2):e127–e138.
60. Costa N, Smits EJ, Kasza J, Salomoni SE, Ferreira M, Hodges PW. Low back pain flares: How do they differ from an increase in pain? *Clin J Pain.* 2021;37(5):313–320.
61. Costa N, Hodges PW, Ferreira ML, Makovey J, Setchell J. What triggers an LBP flare? A content analysis of individuals' perspectives. *Pain Med (Malden, Mass).* 2020;21(1):13–20.
62. LaGraize SC, Borzan J, Peng YB, Fuchs PN. Selective regulation of pain affect following activation of the opioid anterior cingulate cortex system. *Exp Neurol.* 2006;197(1):22–30.
63. Price DD, Von der Gruen A, Miller J, Rafii A, Price C. A psychophysical analysis of morphine analgesia. *Pain.* 1985;22(3):261–269.
64. Oertel BG, Preibisch C, Wallenhorst T, et al. Differential opioid action on sensory and affective cerebral pain processing. *Clin Pharmacol Ther.* 2008;83(4):577–588.
65. Porreca F, Navratilova E. Reward, motivation, and emotion of pain and its relief. *Pain.* 2017;158 Suppl 1:S43–S49.
66. Navratilova E, Porreca F. Reward and motivation in pain and pain relief. *Nature Neurosci.* 2014;17(10):1304–1312.
67. Martel MO, Edwards RR, Jamison RN. The relative contribution of pain and psychological factors to opioid misuse: A 6-month observational study. *Am Psychol.* 2020;75(6):772–783.
68. Carpenter RW, Lane SP, Bruehl S, Trull TJ. Concurrent and lagged associations of prescription opioid use with pain and negative affect in the daily lives of chronic pain patients. *J Consult Clin Psychol.* 2019;87(10):872–886.
69. Colloca L, Lopiano L, Lanotte M, Benedetti F. Overt versus covert treatment for pain, anxiety, and Parkinson's disease. *Lancet Neurol.* 2004;3(11):679–684.

70. Colloca L. The placebo effect in pain therapies. *Ann Rev Pharmacol Toxicol.* 2019;59:191–211.
71. Galaro JK, Celnik P, Chib VS. Motor cortex excitability reflects the subjective value of reward and mediates its effects on incentive-motivated performance. *J Neurosci.* 2019;39(7):1236–1248.
72. Haleem DJ, Nawaz S. Inhibition of reinforcing, hyperalgesic, and motor effects of morphine by buspirone in rats. *J Pain.* 2017;18(1):19–28.
73. Manhapra A, Maclean R, Rosenheck R, Becker W. Are opioids effective analgesics and is physiological opioid dependence benign?: Revising current assumptions to effectively manage long-term opioid therapy and its' deprescribing. 2023. https://doi.org/10.22541/au.169624926.67840172/v1578d01f9e556cd12872ba6567b.pdf.
74. Solomon RL. Recent experiments testing an opponent-process theory of acquired motivation. *Acta Neurobiol Exp (Wars).* 1980;40(1):271–289.
75. Solomon RL, Corbit JD. An opponent process theory of motivation temporal dynamics of affect. *Psychol Rev.* 1974 Mar;81(2):119–145.
76. Solomon RL, Corbit JD. An opponent-process theory of motivation. *Am Econ Rev.* 1978;68(6):12–24.
77. Manhapra A, Arias AJ, Ballantyne JC. The conundrum of opioid tapering in long-term opioid therapy for chronic pain: A commentary. *Subst Abuse.* 2017:1–10.
78. Koob GF. Neurobiology of opioid addiction: Opponent process, hyperkatifeia, and negative reinforcement. *Biol Psychiatry.* 2020;87(1):44–53.
79. Heilig M, Egli M, Crabbe JC, Becker HC. Acute withdrawal, protracted abstinence and negative affect in alcoholism: Are they linked? *Addict Biol.* 2010;15(2):169–184.
80. Agnoli A, Xing G, Tancredi DJ, Magnan E, Jerant A, Fenton JJ. Association of dose tapering with overdose or mental health crisis among patients prescribed long-term opioids. *JAMA.* 2021;326(5):411–419.

10

Future Directions in Pain Management

Implications for Depression and Mental Health

Jane C. Ballantyne, Mark D. Sullivan, and Jeffrey F. Scherrer

10.1 Research to Determine If Treating Depression and Other Psychiatric Disorders to Remission Leads to Safer Opioid Prescribing

As described in this volume, depression, anxiety disorders, and posttraumatic stress disorder (PTSD) are each associated with increased risk for receiving an opioid for non-cancer pain and receiving higher doses and longer-duration prescriptions. While the relationship between these common psychiatric conditions and prescription opioid use has been known for decades, there have been no clinical trials designed to determine if treating these conditions to remission in patients with comorbid chronic pain is followed by less prescription opioid use and lower risk for adverse opioid outcomes such as dependence and overdose.

Research is needed to establish evidence that improvement in these conditions is followed by less pain, decreased opioid use, and improved functioning. Some evidence exists to support the logic of such a clinical trial. The Stepped Care for Affective Disorders and Musculoskeletal Pain (SCAMP) study randomized 250 patients with chronic musculoskeletal pain to either referral for depression treatment versus 12 weeks of antidepressant therapy followed by 6 sessions of pain self-management training and 6 months of follow-up during which treatment was reinforced.[1] The intervention group had significantly greater improvements in depression and pain and improved health-related quality of life at 6- and 12-month follow-ups. However, this study was not intended to assess treatment effects on prescription opioid use. To our knowledge, only one retrospective study evaluated whether adherence to antidepressant treatment enabled opioid cessation. Prior research has demonstrated that patients with depression (with or without pain) who do not adhere to antidepressant medications

---

Jane C. Ballantyne, Mark D. Sullivan, and Jeffrey F. Scherrer, *Future Directions in Pain Management* In: *Pain, the Opioid Epidemic, & Depression.* Edited by: Jeffrey F. Scherrer & Jane C. Ballantyne, Oxford University Press. © Oxford University Press 2024. DOI: 10.1093/9780197675250.003.0010

are less likely to experience improvement,[2] and any response to treatment was markedly lower in nonadherent (56%) versus adherent (83%) patients.[3] Treatment response occurred in 55.8% of patients nonadherent and 82.5% of patients adherent to antidepressant medication. Based on evidence that adherence is a good indicator for likely treatment response, Scherrer and colleagues[4] determined whether patients who develop depression while receiving long-term opioid treatment (LTOT) are more likely to stop opioid use if they adhere to antidepressant medication treatment. The investigators observed adherence to antidepressant medication was associated with a 24% greater likelihood of opioid cessation. It is possible that patients who adhere to antidepressants also adhere to provider instructions about opioid therapy cessation. However, given the robust evidence that antidepressant medication adherence is correlated with treatment response, it is possible that patients who adhered to treatment also experienced relief from depression that in turn enabled opioid cessation. Indeed, preliminary analysis indicates patients who stopped opioid use had a greater reduction in depression symptoms than those who did not.[4]

To our knowledge there are no intervention studies that have determined if screening for and treating depression, anxiety, PTSD, and other conditions associated with poor opioid outcomes reduces risk for LTOT and adverse opioid events such as overdose. A pragmatic trial is needed in which some clinics are randomized to enhanced screening for common psychiatric conditions and aggressive treatment to remission while others remain in care as usual. If it is determined that remission of depression and related conditions is followed by less opioid use, then prescribing guidelines could advise not only screening for these conditions but ensuring that adequate treatment occurs either in tandem or prior to initiating LTOT. This highlights the importance of integrating behavioral health and psychiatry with pain management, as discussed in more detail below.

10.2 Balancing Safe Opioid Prescribing with Access to Pain Management Among Patients with Comorbid Depression

Conceptually, reducing LTOT should mean providing alternatives to opioids for the treatment of chronic pain so that individuals with persistent pain are not driven to seek opioids or can taper off opioids without reemergent pain.

Unfortunately, evidence that alternatives to opioids for pain relief can reduce LTOT is weak.[5] But this is perhaps understandable given that no two patients are alike in either their adoption of opioids or their response to alternative analgesic interventions, making it hard to study this broad question using conventional means of attaining scientific evidence, such as structured comparative trials. Perhaps the more useful question is whether alternatives to opioids, of which there are many, can provide better long-term outcomes in terms of function and quality of life. In this case, the evidence is strongly in favor of alternatives to opioids.[6-8] But our secondary question is whether alternatives to opioids can assist in opioid tapering by providing effective analgesia that could substitute for the opioid over time. Here, the answer is more elusive because opioid tapering in itself is usually painful and the tapering patient often has low expectation that alternative pain-relieving measures will work. Low expectation reduces the efficacy of alternatives to opioids not only in practice, but also in trials.[9,10] However, there is growing evidence that interventions that aid tapering, including multi- or interdisciplinary pain management, can facilitate tapering and that, once off opioids, pain and function are often improved.[11,12] As a general principle, choice of approach needs to be individualized, which sometimes requires trials of therapies and trials of providers until the right match is found. Opioids are best avoided when treating chronic pain, but for the patient already using opioids, treatment needs to be based on optimizing alternative approaches while tapering. Clearly, as already discussed throughout this book, antidepressants may be at the forefront for co-treatment during pain and opioid analgesic management, especially when treating an opioid-dependent patient.

10.3 Care Delivery Models to Increase Safe Opioid Prescribing for Complex Patients with Comorbid Pain and Psychiatric Conditions

10.3.1 Collaborative Care

Collaborative care and integrated behavioral healthcare denote shared care between mental health and primary care providers in the management of pain and mental illness. These care models have been shown to increase the rate of treatment for depression, anxiety, and PTSD.[13] Because most pain treatment occurs in primary care, it is critical that more clinics adopt integrated behavioral healthcare. Integrated behavioral health providers can focus on the psychological and psychosocial needs of the patient, monitor for depression, and initiate psychotherapy to complement psychotropic medications and pain therapies. Another approach to integrated care for patients with pain and comorbid mental illness has been proposed by Goesling and colleagues.[14] Psychiatrists can serve in a consulting role or ideally be integrated into primary care and pain treatment clinics.[14] This is appropriate because primary care physicians and pain providers receive little training in psychiatry, and psychiatrists receive little training in pain management. Failure to treat underlying mental illness will negatively impact pain management. Howe and Sullivan[15] argue that psychiatry should have a central role in our response to the opioid epidemic. Psychiatrists can also manage patients with mood disorders and co-occurring problems with prescription opioids, including opioid use disorder (OUD). Psychiatry can also assist patients who experience distress and unsuccessful opioid tapers by managing worsening symptoms of mood disorder and initiating buprenorphine for risk reduction or to treat OUD. To date, psychiatric research and clinical services for patients with chronic pain have largely been focused on patients with OUD. The significant role played by depression, PTSD, and other mental health disorders in opioid prescribing, opioid risk, and chronic pain outcomes generally argues that psychiatry needs to play a bigger role.

Collaborative care models show promise for safer opioid prescribing and increased access to buprenorphine for OUD.[16] For example, the Veterans Health Administration's (VA) Integrated Pain team involves a collocated medical provider, psychologist, and pharmacists in VA primary care. This new model, compared to usual primary care, resulted in substantially greater opioid dose reduction at 3 and 6 months, and safer prescribing was more often adopted, as indicated by more frequent urine drug screens, naloxone kit distribution, and decreases in benzodiazepine co-medication.[17]

Currently, the majority of patients in the United States do not have access to integrated care. Onwumere et al.[18] argue that studies are needed to determine how to improve integration of care and improve pain management in persons with mental illness. Such efforts will require input from stakeholders including patients, their caregivers, and clinicians. Implementation research is needed to identify barriers and facilitators to expanding effective care integration.[18]

FUTURE DIRECTIONS 169

10.3.2 Whole Health

Recently the U.S. VA launched a Whole Health initiative. The Whole Health system creates an interface between patients' personal health goals, well-being programs, and whole health clinical care in a model incorporating health coaching, health planning, and treatment that aligns with patient goals. For pain, this approach, including complementary and integrative medicine, was shown to lead to a 12% reduction in opioid doses over 1 year, while routine care resulted in a 4% reduction.[19]

10.3.3 Social determinants

It is increasingly recognized that health occurs in the setting of where we live, work, and play. These social determinants of health need to be incorporated into pain management for patients with comorbid mental illness. Social determinants have been shown to be important for back pain prevalence and outcome. For instance, the social environment is associated with odds of receiving a prescription opioid for new back pain encounters.[20] Specifically, patients seen in primary care for a new back pain diagnosis were 80% more likely to receive a prescription opioid if they lived in a low socioeconomic neighborhood, even after controlling for race.[20]

Although we know how social determinants contribute to many health disparities, there is limited evidence on how to change the social and built environment to positively impact the opioid epidemic.[21] Case and Deaton[22,23] have shown that opioid prescribing in the United States is related to various indices of social deprivation, including falling real wages, declining attachment to employment, falling religious participation, and increasing rates of nonmarital childbearing alongside declining rates of marriage. Research is needed to determine if social policies (e.g., crime prevention, increased access to healthcare) impact odds of receiving an opioid for non-cancer pain and modify risk for LTOT and opioid misuse, dependence, and overdose.

The question for medical providers involved in the treatment of pain and depression is how to take our understanding of the critical role of social factors in chronic pain development into the exam room. Are healthcare providers completely powerless in their ability to prevent or minimize the trauma that underlies so much chronic illness or change harmful lifestyles?

Indeed, it may seem a daunting task beyond the control of medicine. Yet there are ways to make inroads into this type of prevention, which begin with recognition and discussion. Although many social issues are difficult for the biomedically trained provider to broach, having the conversation over the course of any enduring relationship between patient and provider is a necessary first step. From the conversation flows intervention, such as psychological support, social support, lifestyle coaching, and simple understanding on the part of the patient of the link between psychosocial factors and pain. One way to overcome negative influences from the environment may be equity-oriented healthcare.[24] It is proposed that, in primary care, chronic pain, mental illness, and exposure to violence often occur together to impact health and quality of life.[24] Equity-oriented care is meant to reduce the impact of social inequalities such as poverty, access to housing, and healthcare. For the disadvantaged, clinics can adopt hours that align with disjointed schedules experienced by the disadvantaged who may have to work multiple jobs to make ends meet. Overcoming negative social determinants of health includes provider engagement and ability to create a safe environment and tailor treatment to the unique needs of the patients' environment. Whether it is policy or clinical practice that reduces the impact of inequalities generated by disparities in social determinants of health, an end to the opioid epidemic will require adopting equity-oriented healthcare.

10.3.4 The Promise of Informatics and Digital Apps

The electronic health record (EHR) has introduced a host of opportunities to improve work flow, documentation, and the application of evidence-based medicine. For instance, providers who have access to automated clinical reminders may be more likely to screen for mental illness prior to initiating opioids when prompted by the EHR to do so. The electronic medical record offers a platform to implement predictive models of high-risk opioid use, risk for mental illness, and opioid misuse and OUD. While numerous machine learning models have been introduced in the literature, much less is known about the implementation and impact of such tools in daily clinical practice. A meaningful exception is the VA's implementation of an opioid safety initiative that uses an electronic dashboard that contains patients' relevant clinical data and opioid-related prescribing information on risky prescribing such as dual benzodiazepine–high-dose opioid prescriptions.[25] The dashboard alerts providers to risky prescriptions and prompts them to take appropriate risk reduction actions.[25] In the year following implementation of the dash-board, there was a 16% decrease in high-dose (>100 morphine milligram equivalent [MME]) opioid prescriptions.[25] Outside the VA, prescription monitoring, which documents filled controlled substance prescriptions, can be accessed by providers in their own state. Prescription monitoring can be accessed within some but not all EHRs.

Digital apps have the potential to assist patients with pain management, depression, and opioid use problems. Digital therapeutics include prescription and non-prescription mobile medical apps, mobile health apps, virtual reality, and tele-medicine.[26] Digital therapeutics offer treatment complementary to standard clinical practice and provide patient-centered care because apps are designed to be adaptive to patient characteristics. It is possible that such digital apps will increase access to non-opioid pain management and reduce risky opioid use. For instance, "BackRx" is a mobile app for discogenic low back pain that delivers virtual yoga and Pilates exercises.[26] Apps are also approved by the U.S. Food and Drug Administration as adjunct therapy for buprenorphine treatment in OUD (e.g., RESET-0). Such apps have shown improvement in therapy and cost effectiveness.[27]

10.4 Investing to End the Opioid Epidemic

Simulations project only a 0.3% reduction in fatal prescription opioid overdoses assuming reductions in prescribing, but, in combination with increased access to naloxone and treatment expansion, the projected decrease in fatal opioid overdoses over 10 years rises to 37%.[28] A major National Institutes of Health investment, the HEAL Initiative, holds promise for reducing the impacts of the opioid epidemic. Goldstein and colleagues[21] propose HEAL's success will need investment in (1) risk identification; (2) intervention development; (3) social determinants, health equity, and policy; and, last, (4) dissemination. With increased funding for precision medicine, we should expect to see research developments designed to prevent adverse opioid outcomes in high-risk patients with comorbid psychiatric disorders. This patient population will continue to experience a disproportionate burden of the opioid epidemic until potential interventions are developed for them. Identification of high-risk patients and targeting of these patients for comprehensive pain treatment may provide our best means of preventing adverse outcomes from opioids. Supportive interdisciplinary treatment may be effective enough that opioids can be avoided. Such treatment is also the best option for people already on opioids having difficulty tapering and for the small minority of patients judged suitable for opioid treatment.

While it is well established that patients with pain and comorbid depression, anxiety, and PTSD are more likely to receive LTOT than those without these conditions, the mechanisms behind this relationship remain unknown. Increased non-medical opioid use has been suggested as a mechanism leading to OUD in patients with depression. In addition to experiencing less analgesia, short-term euphoria may be mistaken by patients as relief from depression.[29] Studies are needed that can discern different motives for continued prescription opioid use in persons with versus without comorbid psychiatric conditions. By understanding unique factors contributing to LTOT in persons with these conditions, interventions can be tailored to patients with comorbid mental illness. Further understanding of the endogenous opioid system in pain and depression may yield novel therapies. Increased buprenorphine access is another area where medication targets both mood disorder and reduces pain and opioid craving. Reducing depression can improve pain and reduce risk for adverse opioid events such as overdose.[29]

References

1. Kroenke K, Bair MJ, Damush TM, et al. Optimized antidepressant therapy and pain self-management in primary care patients with depression and musculoskeletal pain: A randomized controlled trial. *JAMA.* 2009;301(20):2099–2110.
2. Ho SC, Chong HY, Chaiyakunapruk N, Tangiisuran B, Jacob SA. Clinical and economic impact of non-adherence to antidepressants in major depressive disorder: A systematic review. *J Affect Disord.* 2016;193:1–10.
3. Akerblad AC, Bengtsson F, von Knorring L, Ekselius L. Response, remission and relapse in relation to adherence in primary care treatment of depression: A 2-year outcome study. *Int Clin Psychopharmacol.* 2006;21(2):117–124.
4. Scherrer JF, Salas J, Sullivan MD, et al. Impact of adherence to antidepressants on long-term prescription opioid use cessation. *Br J Psychiatry.* 2018;212(2):103–111.
5. Avery N, McNeilage AG, Stanaway F, et al. Efficacy of interventions to reduce long term opioid treatment for chronic non-cancer pain: systematic review and meta-analysis. *BMJ.* 2022;377:e066375.
6. Chou R, Hartung D, Turner J, et al. AHRQ Comparative Effectiveness Reviews. In: *Opioid Treatments for Chronic Pain.* Agency for Healthcare Research and Quality (US); 2020.
7. Krebs EE, Gravely A, Nugent S, et al. Effect of opioid vs nonopioid medications on pain-related function in patients with chronic back pain or hip or knee osteoarthritis pain: The SPACE randomized clinical trial. *JAMA.* 2018;319(9):872–882.
8. Jones CM, Lin CC, Day RO, et al. OPAL: A randomised, placebo-controlled trial of opioid analgesia for the reduction of pain severity in people with acute spinal pain: A statistical analysis plan. *Trials.* 2022;23(1):212.
9. Langford DJ, Lou R, Sheen S, et al. Expectations for improvement: A neglected but potentially important covariate or moderator for chronic pain clinical trials. *J Pain.* 2023;24(4):575–581.

FUTURE DIRECTIONS 173

10. Rosenkjær S, Lunde SJ, Kirsch I, Vase L. Expectations: How and when do they contribute to placebo analgesia? *Front Psychiatry*. 2022;13:817179.
11. Sandhu HK, Booth K, Furlan AD, et al. Reducing opioid use for chronic pain with a group-based intervention: A randomized clinical trial. *JAMA*. 2023;329(20):1745–1756.
12. Sullivan MD, Turner JA, DiLodovico C, D'Appollonio A, Stephens K, Chan YF. Prescription opioid taper support for outpatients with chronic pain: A randomized controlled trial. *J Pain*. 2017;18(3):308–318.
13. Woltmann E, Grogan-Kaylor A, Perron B, Georges H, Kilbourne AM, Bauer MS. Comparative effectiveness of collaborative chronic care models for mental health conditions across primary, specialty, and behavioral health care settings: Systematic review and meta-analysis. *Am J Psychiatry*. 2012;169(8):790–804.
14. Goesling J, Lin LA, Clauw DJ. Psychiatry and pain management: At the intersection of chronic pain and mental health. *Curr Psychiatry Rep*. 2018;20(2):12.
15. Howe CQ, M.D. S. The missing "p" in pain management: How the current opioid epidemic highlights the need for psychiatric services in chronic pain care. *Gen Hosp Psychiatry*. 2014;36(1):99–104.
16. Heavey SC, Bleasdale J, Rosenfeld EA, Beehler GP. Collaborative care models to improve pain and reduce opioid use in primary care: A systematic review. *J Gen Intern Med*. 2023 Oct;38(13):3021–3040.
17. Seal KH, Rife T, Li Y, Gibson C, Tighe J. Opioid reduction and risk mitigation in VA primary care: Outcomes from the integrated pain team initiative. *J Gen Intern Med*. 2020;35(4):1238–1244.
18. Onwumere J, Stubbs B, Stirling M, et al. Pain management in people with severe mental illness: An agenda for progress. *Pain*. 2022;163(9):1653–1660.
19. Zeliadt SB, Douglas JH, Gelman H, et al. Effectiveness of a whole health model of care emphasizing complementary and integrative health on reducing opioid use among patients with chronic pain. *BMC Health Serv Res*. 2022;22(1):1053.
20. Gebauer S, Salas J, Scherrer JF. Neighborhood socioeconomic status and receipt of opioid medication for new back pain diagnosis. *J Am Board Fam Med*. 2017;30(6):775–783.
21. Goldstein AB, Oudekerk BA, Blanco C. HEAL Preventing opioid use disorder: A vision for research to increase access to prevention services. *Prev Sci*. 2023 Oct;24(Suppl 1):8–15.
22. Case A, Deaton A. Rising morbidity and mortality in midlife among white non-Hispanic Americans in the 21st century. *Proc Natl Acad Sci U S A*. 2015;112(49):15078–15083.
23. Case A, Deaton A. The great divide: Education, despair, and death. *Annu Rev Econ*. 2022:1–21.
24. Ford-Gilboe M, Wathen CN, Varcoe C, et al. How equity-oriented health care affects health: Key mechanisms and implications for primary health care practice and policy. *Milbank Q*. 2018;96(4):635–671.
25. Lin LA, Bohnert ASB, Kerns RD, Clay MA, Ganoczy D, Ilgen MA. Impact of the Opioid Safety Initiative on opioid-related prescribing in veterans. *Pain*. 2017;158(5):833–839.
26. Rohaj A, Bulaj G. Digital therapeutics (DTx) expand multimodal treatment options for chronic low back pain: The nexus of precision medicine, patient education, and public health. *Healthcare (Basel)*. 2023;11(10):1469.
27. Giravi HY, Biskupiak Z, Tyler LS, Bulaj G. Adjunct digital interventions improve opioid-based pain management: Impact of virtual reality and mobile applications on patient-centered pharmacy care. *Front Digit Health*. 2022;4:884047.
28. Ballreich J, Mansour O, Hu E, et al. Modeling mitigation strategies to reduce opioid-related morbidity and mortality in the US. *JAMA Netw Open*. 2020;3(11):e2023677.
29. Sullivan MD. Depression effects on long-term prescription opioid use, abuse, and addiction. *Clin J Pain*. 2018;34(9):878–884.

Index

For the benefit of digital users, indexed terms that span two pages (e.g., 52–53) may, on occasion, appear on only one of those pages.

Figures and tables are indicated by *f* and *t* following the page number.

Abstinence syndrome, 157–58
ACC (anterior cingulated cortex), 16
acceptance and commitment therapy (ACT), 63, 64*t*, 67, 68
acetaminophen, 87
ACTH (adrenocorticotropic hormone), 15
acute pain, 29–30, 38
  definition of, 6
  healthcare access and quality and, 123
addiction, drug, 140
adjuvant pain medications, 86
adrenocorticotropic hormone (ACTH), 15
agoraphobia, 81–82
allostasis, 141, 157–58
allostatic opponent effect, 157–58
allostatic theory of drug-seeking behavior, 141
American Academy of Sleep Medicine Standards of Practice Committee, 91
amitriptyline, 86–87
amygdala, 16
androgen deficiency, 55–56
anhedonia, 18–19, 53
anterior cingulated cortex (ACC), 16
anti-reward system, 152
anticonvulsants, 86–87, 91, 95
antidepressants, 86, 91, 165–66
antiepileptic medications, 95
antihistamines, 86
antipsychotics, 86, 91, 98, 101–2
anxiety
  with chronic pain, 4, 62, 80–88
  as homeostatic emotion, 2–3, 29
  prevalence of, 82
anxiety disorders
  prevalence of, 80–81, 82
  psychological vulnerabilities, 83
  treatment of, 86
Asian patients, 71
Assyrians, 149
autonomic nervous system (ANS), 23–24

Avicenna, 149
azapirones, 86

back pain, 25, 140
  BackRx app for, 171
  chronic, 30, 81, 83, 86–87
BackRx app, 171
barriers to care, 72
BD. *See* bipolar disorder
behavioral activation, 65–66
behavioral drive, 22–23, 23*f*
benzodiazepines, 86, 87, 91, 101–2
bias by indication, 40, 41*f*
  controlling for, 41
bias toward BIPOC and other minorities, 127–28
biological mechanisms, 55
biopsychosocial concept of pain, 64–65
bipolar disorder (BD), 80, 93–96
Black, Indigenous, and people of color (BIPOC), 71, 127–28, 129
body scan, 66
brain
  pain matrix, 25
  pain perception, 25
  salience network, 25
brief interventions, 69–70
built environment, 125–27
buprenorphine, 6, 125, 145
  adjunct therapy, 171
  for depression, 149
  for depression in LTOT, 5, 148, 155, 158–60
  for depression in opioid dependence, 4–5, 158–60
  for depression in OUD, 154, 171
  future research directions, 145
  guidelines for use of, 145, 148–49
  history of therapeutic use of, 149
  long-term therapy with, 39
  low-dose, 153
  for non-cancer pain, 6
  pharmacology of, 152
  for treatment-refractory depression, 153

176 INDEX

buprenorphine/naloxone, 92, 158–60
buprenorphine/samidorphan, 153–54
bupropion, 87
buspirone, 86

Canadian Community Health Survey, 119–20
cannabis, 95, 101
Cannon, Walter, 23–24
care delivery models, 167–70
Cassell, Eric, 33–34
catastrophizing, 28–29, 63, 64–65
causation, 54
CBT. See cognitive-behavioral therapy
CDC. See Centers for Disease Control and
    Prevention
Centers for Disease Control and Prevention
    (CDC)
  guidelines for prescribing opioids, 6–7, 10,
    123–24, 138–39, 143–44, 148–49
  recommended management strategy for
    when harms outweigh benefits of LTOT,
    155
central pain conditions, 86–87
chronic morphine use, 17
chronic opioid use
  definition of, 7, 39
  hedonic capacity related to, 18
  neuroanatomical changes in, 18
  See also long-term opioid therapy (LTOT);
    opioid use disorder
chronic pain, 38, 62–63
  in anxiety (see chronic pain and anxiety)
  barriers to care, 72
  in bipolar disorder (see chronic pain and
    bipolar disorder)
  CBT strategies for, 65–66
  definition of, 6, 140
  in depression, 5, 7–8, 13, 63–67, 68–72, 148,
    155, 160
  education access and quality and, 122
  guidelines on opioid use for, 148–49
  healthcare access and quality and, 123
  long-term opioid therapy (LTOT) for, 5, 148,
    155–57, 160
  mindfulness strategies for, 66
  neighborhood and environment and, 126
  neurophysiology of, 15, 30–31
  opioid-induced chronic pain syndrome
    (OICP), 139, 156, 158
  prevalence of, 93
  in psychiatric disorders, 80–81, 102
  psychological interventions for, 65–66, 67,
    68–72
  psychological vulnerabilities, 83

in PTSD (see chronic pain and PTSD)
risk factors for, 7–8
in schizophrenia (see chronic pain and
    schizophrenia)
in sleep disorders, 81
chronic pain and anxiety, 4, 62, 80–81
  clinical assessment of, 84
  epidemiology of, 81
  impact on clinical outcomes, 83
  non-pharmacological management of, 88
  opioid therapy in, 87
  pharmacological treatment of, 86
chronic pain and bipolar disorder, 80
  epidemiology of, 93
  impact on clinical outcomes, 94
  non-pharmacological management of, 96
  opioid therapy in, 96
  pharmacological management of, 95
chronic pain and PTSD, 80
  clinical assessment of, 90
  epidemiology of, 88
  impact on clinical outcomes, 90
  non-pharmacological management of, 92
  opioid therapy in, 91
  pharmacological management of, 91
chronic pain and schizophrenia, 80
  clinical assessment of, 99
  epidemiology of, 97
  impact on clinical outcomes, 99
  non-pharmacological management of, 102
  opioid therapy in, 101
  pharmacological treatment of, 100
chronic prescription opioid use, 18. See also
    chronic opioid use
Clinician Administered PTSD Scale for DSM-5
    (CAPS-5), 90–91
co-analgesics, 86
codeine
  drug interactions, 87
  long-term therapy with, 39
  morphine milligram equivalents (MMEs),
    6–7, 40
  for non-cancer pain, 6
cognitive behavioral mediation hypothesis,
    13–14
cognitive-behavioral therapy (CBT), 63, 64
  for chronic pain, 92–93, 96–97
  components, 64t
  to reduce opioid use, 68
  trauma-focused, 92
cognitive processing therapy (CPT), 92
cohort studies
  prospective, 49
  retrospective, 45–48, 47f

collaborative care, 144–45, 167
common pathogenetic mechanisms hypothesis, 13–14
community context, 127–29
comorbidity studies, 82–83
complex persistent opioid dependence (CPOD), 4–5, 156
  behavioral manifestations of, 141
  definition of, 139
  future research directions, 144–45
confounding factors
  controlling for, 41
  pain as, 40–41
connectedness, 127–29
consequence hypothesis, 13–14
Consortium to Study Opioid Risks and Trends (CONSORT), 39
corticosteroids, 15
COVID-19 public health emergency, 125
CPOD. *See* complex persistent opioid dependence
CPT (cognitive processing therapy), 92
CPT (Current Procedural Terminology), 45
Craig, Bud, 22–23
cross-sectional studies, 44
Current Procedural Terminology (CPT), 45

Damasio, Antonio, 23–24
Dawes, Daniel, 129–30
deaths of despair, 127–28
deep TMS, 102
delta opioid receptor (DOR), 16–17, 32, 152
dependence. *See* opioid dependence
depression
  biological mechanisms, 55
  in chronic pain, 7–8, 13, 62–67, 68–72
  definition of, 2–3
  economic stability and, 120
  education access and quality and, 122
  future directions in pain management and, 165
  future research directions, 165
  healthcare access and quality and, 124
  as homeostatic emotion, 29
  incident, 54
  liability for, 54
  in long-term opioid therapy (LTOT), 3, 5, 10, 32–33, 48, 50–51, 51*f*, 53, 54–57, 142, 155–57, 165–66
  in long-term opioid therapy (LTOT) dependence, 148, 160
  in LTOT dependence-induced OICP, 158
  major depressive disorder (MDD), 149
  major depressive episodes, 53

  management of, 68
  neighborhood and environment and, 126
  neurophysiology of, 13–14, 16, 30–31
  new-onset, 45, 51, 56, 57
  in opioid dependence, 142
  in opioid epidemic, 7
  in opioid taper, 142
  in opioid use, 32–33, 68, 142
  in opioid use disorder, 52, 154
  pain, depression, opioid cycle, 10*f*, 10–11
  in pain, 3, 7–8, 13–14, 62
  pain management in, 166
  prescription opioids and, 9, 37
  protective mechanisms against, 129
  psychological interventions for, 68–72
  psychosocial mechanisms, 56
  risk, 37
  risk factors, 10
  safe opioid prescribing in, 166
  social, community context, and connectedness and, 128
  social and structural determinants of health and, 117, 129
  treatment of, 149–51, 153–55, 165
  treatment-refractory, 150–51, 153, 155
deQuincey, Thomas, 150
desipramine, 86–87
Diagnostic and Statistical Manual of Mental Disorders, 139
diathesis-stress model, 13–14
digital apps, 171
dihydrocodeine, 6, 39
dopamine, 14
DOR (delta opioid receptor), 16–17, 32, 152
dosage
  considerations for standardizing, 40
  escalating dose, 51
dose, 6–7
drug addiction, 140
Drug Enforcement Agency, 6
drug interactions, 87
drug-seeking behavior, 141
duloxetine, 86–87
dynorphin, 18–19

e-values, 46–47
EAET (emotional awareness and expression therapy), 31–32
economic stability, 118–20
ECT (electroconvulsive therapy), 97
education access and quality, 121–22
educational programs, 123
electroconvulsive therapy (ECT), 97
electronic health records (EHRs), 170–71

178 INDEX

EMDR (eye movement desensitization and reprocessing), 92
emotion(s)
  homeostatic, 22, 27, 29
  James-Lange theory of, 23–24
emotional awareness and expression therapy (EAET), 31–32
emotional pain, 18–19
endorphins, 140, 150
enkephalins, 140
environmental conditions, 125–27
equity-oriented care, 169–70
experimental pain, 97–98
explain pain model, 31–32
eye movement desensitization and reprocessing (EMDR), 92

family risk factors, 127
fentanyl, 6, 39
fibromyalgia, 81, 83, 86–87, 140
financial investment, 171
financial literacy, 121–22
fMRI (functional magnetic resonance imaging), 16, 30
food insecurity, 119–20
frequency of use, escalating, 51
functional magnetic resonance imaging (fMRI), 16, 30
future directions
  in pain management, 165
  in research, 71–72, 102, 143, 165, 172

GABA (gamma-aminobutyric acid), 17
gabapentin, 86–87, 95
GAD-2, 85
GAD-7, 85
Galen, 149
gamma-aminobutyric acid (GABA), 17
gate control theory of pain, 64–65
generalized anxiety disorder, 81–82, 83
gray matter, 18
guided imagery, 66

HADS (Hospital Anxiety and Depression Scale), 85
haloperidol, 98
HCSRN (Health Care System Research Network), 45
HEAL Initiative (NIH), 171–72
health-promoting environments, 126
healthcare access and quality, 123–25
Health Care System Research Network (HCSRN), 45

health insurance, 124
health literacy, 121
Healthy People 2030, 118, 121
hedonic capacity, 18
Henry Ford Health system, 45
heroin, 33
hippocampus, 16
Hippocrates, 149
Hispanic patients, 71
home environment, 126–27
homeostatic view, 22, 27, 29
Homer, 149
Hospital Anxiety and Depression Scale (HADS), 85
housing, 118–19, 120–21
HPA (hypothalamic-pituitary-adrenal) axis, 15, 18
hurt, pain and, 28, 33
hydrocodone
  drug interactions, 87
  long-term therapy with, 39
  morphine milligram equivalents (MMEs), 6–7, 40
  for non-cancer pain, 6
hydromorphone, 6, 39
hydroxyzine, 86
hyperalgesia, 55
hyperarousal, 89
hyperkatifeia, 52, 140–41
hypothalamic-pituitary-adrenal (HPA) axis, 15, 18

ICD (International Classification of Diseases), 45, 46, 139
illicit opioid use, 53
imagery, guided, 66
imperative theory of pain, 24
informatics, 170
insomnia, 55, 89
instrumental variables, 54
Integrated Pain teams (VHA), 168
interdisciplinary pain programs
  future research directions, 144–45
  during opioid taper, 142
interleukin-1, 15
interleukin-6, 15
International Classification of Diseases (ICD), 45, 46, 139
inverse probability of treatment weighting (IPTW), 42, 43f
irritable bowel syndrome, 81, 83

Kaiser Permanente, 45
kappa opioid receptor (KOR), 16–17, 18–19, 32, 151–52

INDEX 179

ketamine, 101
key concepts, 5–6
Klein, Colin, 24, 27, 28–29
KOR (kappa opioid receptor), 16–17, 18–19, 32, 151–52

lamina I spino-thalamo-cortical system, 22–23, 23f
lateral orbital prefrontal cortex (LOPFC), 16
levorphanol, 6, 39
LGBTQ population, 127–28
lithium, 87
long-term opioid therapy (LTOT), 145
  definition of, 7, 39
  depression with, 3, 5, 10, 32–33, 48, 50–51, 51f, 53, 54–57, 142, 148, 155–57, 160, 165–66
  effects of, 32–33, 53, 55
  endogenous opioid interactions, 32
  future research directions, 143–44, 165–66
  pain with, 157
  risks and associated harms, 138–39
  selection of patients for, 57, 155
  side effects, 53
long-term opioid therapy (LTOT) dependence, 148, 160. See also opioid dependence
long-term opioid therapy (LTOT) dependence-induced OICP, 158
LOPFC (lateral orbital prefrontal cortex), 16
low back pain, 25, 140
  BackRx app for, 171
  chronic, 30, 81, 83, 86–87
LTOT. See long-term opioid therapy

magnetic resonance imaging (MRI), 25
  functional (fMRI), 16, 30
major depressive disorder (MDD), 149
major depressive episodes, 53
McGill Pain Questionnaire, 21–22
MDD (major depressive disorder), 149
medial dorsal nucleus, ventral caudal part (MDvc), 22–23
Melzack, Ronald, 21–22
mental health, 62–63
meperidine, 6, 39
methadone, 6, 39, 125
migraine headaches, 81, 93–94
milnacipran, 86–87
mindfulness, 63, 64t, 66, 68
mindfulness-based stress reduction, 66
minority populations, 127–28
mirtazapine, 86

MMEs (morphine milligram equivalents), 6–7, 40
mood disorders
  in chronic pain, 62
  risk of, 50–51, 51f
mood stabilizers, 91
MOR (mu opioid receptor), 16–17, 32, 148–49, 151–52
morphine
  long-term therapy with, 39, 158–60
  mechanism of action, 17
  for non-cancer pain, 6
morphine milligram equivalents (MMEs), 6–7, 40
morphinism, 150
MRI. See magnetic resonance imaging
mu opioid receptor (MOR), 16–17, 32, 148–49, 151–52

naltrexone, 125
National Comorbidity Survey Part II, 81–82, 89
National Epidemiologic Survey on Alcohol and Related Conditions, 95
National Institute of Health (NIH)
  HEAL Initiative, 171–72
  "Pain Assessment Resources for Professionals," 84–85
neighborhood and built environment, 125–27
neuropathic pain
  definition of, 140
  pharmacological treatment of, 86–87, 95
neurophysiology, 13–14, 19, 56
New England Journal of Medicine, 25
new users, 47
new user studies, 7
New York Times, 33
NIH. See National Institute of Health
nociceptin/orphanin FQ (NOP) receptors, 152
nociceptive pain, 140
nociplastic pain, 140
non-cancer pain
  chronic, 6 (see also chronic pain)
  measuring, 38
  overview, 7
  types of opioids prescribed for, 6
nonsteroidal antiinflammatory drugs (NSAIDs), 87
NOP (nociceptin/orphanin FQ) receptors, 152
norepinephrine, 14
nortriptyline, 86–87
NSAIDs (nonsteroidal antiinflammatory drugs), 87

180 INDEX

obsessive-compulsive disorder, 83
OICP (opioid-induced chronic pain
    syndrome), 139, 156, 157–58
Operation Enduring Freedom, 89
Operation Iraqi Freedom, 89
opioid cessation programs, 68
opioid dependence
    buprenorphine treatment of, 4–5, 148, 160
    complex persistent (CPOD), 4–5, 139, 141,
        144–45, 156
    definition of, 139
    depression with chronic pain and, 5
    LTOT dependence-induced OICP, 157–58
    physiologic, 139
    refractory, 139
opioid epidemic
    investing to end, 171
    overview, 8
opioid-induced chronic pain syndrome
    (OICP), 139, 156, 157–58
    LTOT dependence-induced, 158
opioid medications. *See* prescription opioids
opioid misuse, 53. *See also* opioid use disorder
    (OUD)
opioid receptors, 16–17
opioids
    endogenous, 16–17, 32, 140
    exogenous, 13
    illicit, 53
    medications (*see* prescription opioids)
opioid taper, 4–5, 145, 155
    depression in, 142
    future research directions, 143–45
    interdisciplinary pain treatment during, 142
opioid therapy. *See* prescription opioids
opioid use
    chronic, 7, 18, 39 (*see also* long-term opioid
        therapy; opioid use disorder)
    depression in, 32–33, 68, 142
    effects of misuse, 53
    hedonic capacity related to, 18
    illicit, 53
    management of, 68
    neuroanatomical changes in, 18
opioid use disorder (OUD)
    buprenorphine treatment of, 171
    depression in, 52, 154
    economic stability and, 120
    education access and quality and, 122
    healthcare access and quality and, 125
    neighborhood and environment and, 127
    psychosocial mechanisms, 56
    risk factors for, 127
    risk for depression and, 52

social, community context, and
    connectedness and, 129
social and structural determinants of health
    and, 117, 129
opium, 149–50
Opium cure *(Opiumkur),* 150
opponent process theory, 140
organizational health literacy, 121
OUD. *See* opioid use disorder
oxycodone
    long-term therapy with, 39
    morphine milligram equivalents (MMEs),
        6–7, 40
    for non-cancer pain, 6
oxymorphone, 6, 39

pacing, 65–66
PAG (periaqueductal gray), 15
pain, 2–3, 140
    acute, 6, 29–30, 38, 123
    back, 25, 30
    biopsychosocial concept of, 64–65
    breakthrough, 39–40
    central, 86–87
    chronic (*see* chronic pain)
    clinical, 24–25
    definition of, 6, 13
    with depression, 3, 7–8, 13–14, 62–67, 68
    economic stability and, 119
    education access and quality and, 122
    emotional, 18–19
    experimental, 97–98
    gate control theory of, 64–65
    as homeostatic emotion, 22, 29
    with hurt and suffering, 28, 33
    intuitive ideas about, 21
    as key confounding factor, 40–41
    Klein's imperative theory of, 24
    with long-term opioid therapy (LTOT), 157
    measuring, 38
    medically unexplained, 24–25
    modulation of, 15
    motivational forces of, 28–29
    neighborhood and environment and, 126
    neuropathic, 86–87, 95, 140
    neurophysiological mechanisms, 13–14
    nociceptive, 140
    nociplastic, 140
    non-cancer, 6, 7, 38
    with opioid use, 68
    perception of, 25
    postoperative, 86–87
    prescription opioids for, 6–7
    with psychiatric conditions, 167–70

INDEX 181

psychological interventions for, 67
psychosocial factors, 80
purpose of, 26
sensory properties of, 21–22
sleep and, 80
social, community context, and
  connectedness and, 128
social and structural determinants of health
  and, 129
with tissue damage, 21
pain, depression, opioid cycle, 10f, 10–11
Pain and Opioids IN Treatment (POINT)
  study, 44, 50–51
Pain Anxiety Symptoms Scale, 85
pain assessment, 99–100
"Pain Assessment Resources for Professionals"
  (NIH Pain Consortium), 84–85
pain catastrophizing, 63
Pain Catastrophizing Scale, 63
pain interference, 56, 62–63, 84–85
pain management
  barriers to care, 72
  care delivery models, 167–70
  CBT strategies, 64–66
  challenges and potential solutions, 68
  in depression, 166
  future directions, 165
  interdisciplinary programs, 142
  long-term (see long-term opioid therapy)
  mindfulness strategies, 66
  in psychiatric conditions, 167–70
  psychological interventions, 68–72
  safe opioid prescribing for complex patients,
    167–70
pain matrix, 25
pain neuroscience education (PNE), 31–32
pain relief, 33–34
pain reprocessing therapy (PRT), 31–32,
  64–65
pain severity, 62–63, 71
panic disorder, 81–83
paroxetine, 87, 91
Patient Health Questionnaire 8-item
  (PHQ-8), 44
Patient-Reported Outcomes Measurement
  Information System (PROMIS) measures,
  84–85
PCL (PTSD Checklist), 46
peer recovery support, 129
PEG-3, 84–85
pentazocine, 6, 39
periaqueductal gray (PAG), 15
personal health literacy, 121
PFC (prefrontal cortex), 16

pharmacological treatment
  of chronic pain and anxiety, 86
  of chronic pain and bipolar disorder, 95
  of chronic pain and PTSD, 91
  of chronic pain and schizophrenia, 100
  See also specific medications
PHQ-8 (Patient Health Questionnaire
  8-item), 44
physical activity, 65–66
physical nociception, 140
physiologic dependence, 139. See also opioid
  dependence
Pilates, 171
placebo effects, 157
PNE (pain neuroscience education), 31–32
POINT (Pain and Opioids IN Treatment)
  study, 44, 50–51
policy, 72
political determinants of health, 129–30
poppy (Papaver somniferum), 149
postoperative pain, 86–87
posttraumatic stress disorder (PTSD), 30–31,
  32–33, 83
  chronic pain and, 80, 88–92
  diagnostic codes for, 46
  treatment of, 92
prazosin, 91
prefrontal cortex (PFC), 16
pregabalin, 86–87, 95
prescription monitoring, 170–71
prescription opioids
  adverse effects, 10, 17
  CDC guidelines, 6–7, 10, 123–24, 138–39,
    143–44
  chronic use of, 18, 67
  dependence on (see opioid dependence)
  for depression, 150
  depression with, 9, 17, 44, 56
  dosage, 40
  dose, 6–7
  duration of use, 6–7
  escalating dose and frequency of
    use, 51
  frequency of use, 6
  future research directions, 143–44, 165
  guidelines on use of, 148–49
  liability for greater use of, 54
  long-acting formulations, 6
  long-term (see long-term opioid therapy)
  measures, 6
  mechanism of action, 16, 140
  new users, 47
  for non-cancer pain, 6
  overdose deaths due to, 1

182 INDEX

prescription opioids (*cont.*)
pain, depression, opioid cycle, 10*f*, 10–11
for pain, 6–7
for pain and anxiety, 87
for pain and bipolar disorder, 96
for pain and depression, 68, 166
for pain and PTSD, 91
for pain and schizophrenia, 101
prescribing rates, 1, 138
psychological interventions to reduce use of, 67
for PTSD, 91–92
risk of depression with, 37
risk of incident mood disorder with, 50–51, 51*f*
safe prescribing, 166
selection of patients for, 57
short-acting formulations, 6
social and structural determinants of health and, 117, 129
Prescription Opioids and Depression Pathways Cohort study, 57–58
Price, Don, 21
primary care, 69–70
progressive muscle relaxation, 66
prolonged exposure (PE), 92
PROMIS (Patient-Reported Outcomes Measurement Information System) measures, 84–85
propensity scores (PS), 41, 42
prospective cohort studies, 49
protracted withdrawal/abstinence syndrome, 157–58
PRT (pain reprocessing therapy), 31–32, 64–65
PS (propensity scores), 41, 42
psychiatric disorders
chronic pain and, 80–81, 102
future research direction, 165
medically unexplained pain and, 24–25
safe opioid prescribing for complex patients with pain and, 167–70
treatment of, 165
psychoeducation, 64–65
psychological treatment
changes in depression and pain with, 62
interventions for chronic pain and depression, 63–67, 64*t*, 68–72
to reduce prescription opioid use among individuals with chronic pain, 67
psychopathology, 53
psychosis, 101
psychosocial factors, 80
psychosocial mechanisms, 56

PTSD (posttraumatic stress disorder), 30–31, 32–33
PTSD Checklist (PCL), 46
PTSD checklist for DSM-5 (PCL-5), 90–91
public health, 57

quetiapine, 91

racism, 127–28
refractory dependence, 139. *See also* opioid dependence
relaxation
CBT strategy, 65
progressive muscle relaxation, 66
research directions, 71–72, 102, 143, 165, 172
research gaps, 102
retrospective cohort studies
design, 47*f*, 47
evidence from, 48
results from, 45
strengths and weaknesses of, 45
reward deficiency, 18–19
Ryan-Haight Act, 125

safe prescribing
for complex patients, 167–70
in depression, 166
salience network, 25
SCAMP (Stepped Care for Affective Disorders and Musculoskeletal Pain) study, 165–66
scar hypothesis, 13–14
Schedule II medications, 6
Schedule III medications, 6
Schedule IV medications, 6
schizophrenia, 80, 97–102
SCID (Structured Clinical Interview for DSM-IV), 46
SDOH (social determinants of health), 4, 118, 119*f*, 169
sedating antipsychotics, 101–2
sedative hypnotics, 91–92
selective serotonin reuptake inhibitors (SSRIs), 81, 86–87, 91
serotonin, 14
serotonin-norepinephrine reuptake inhibitors (SNRIs), 86–87, 91
sleep disturbances, 46
with chronic pain, 81, 94
PTSD-related, 89, 91
SNRIs (serotonin-norepinephrine reuptake inhibitors), 86–87, 91
social and community context and connectedness, 127–29

social and structural determinants of health (SSDOH), 117, 129
social anxiety disorder, 81–82
social determinants of health (SDOH), 4, 118, 119f, 169
social media, 128
social participation, 127–28
Solomon, Richard, 140–41
somatic marker hypothesis, 23–24
Spielberger State Trait Anxiety Inventory, 85
SSDOH (social and structural determinants of health), 117, 129
SSRIs (selective serotonin reuptake inhibitors), 81, 86–87, 91
standardized mean difference, 42
Stepped Care for Affective Disorders and Musculoskeletal Pain (SCAMP) study, 165–66
stigma, 127–28
stress, 13–14
Structured Clinical Interview for DSM-IV (SCID), 46
substance use disorders (SUDs), 92, 117, 127, 129
suffering
    definition of, 33–34
    pain and, 28, 33

tapentadol, 6, 39
TCAs. *See* tricyclic antidepressants
telemedicine, 69–71
Thriving Together: A Springboard for Equitable Recovery and Resilience in Communities Across America, 129–30
tissue damage, 21
TMS (transcranial magnetic stimulation), 97, 102
tramadol, 6, 39, 87
transcranial magnetic stimulation (TMS), 97, 102
transgender population, 127–28
trauma-focused CBT, 92
treatment courts, 129

treatment-refractory depression (TRD), 150–51, 153, 155
treatment weighting, inverse probability of (IPTW), 42, 43f
tricyclic antidepressants (TCAs), 86–87, 91, 95

U.S. Department of Defense (DoD), 148–49
U.S. Department of Health and Human Services (HHS)
    guidelines for buprenorphine use, 145
    guidelines for prescribing opioids, 148–49
    Healthy People 2030, 118, 121
U.S. Department of Veterans Affairs (VA)
    guidelines for opioid use for chronic pain, 148–49
    opioid safety initiative, 170–71
    Whole Health initiative, 169
U.S. Food and Drug Administration (FDA), 86–87, 125, 171
U.S. Veterans Health Administration (VHA), 8, 45, 48
    Integrated Pain teams, 168

vagus nerve stimulation (VNS), 97
values-based action, 67
venlafaxine, 86–87, 91
ventral medial nucleus, posterior (VMpo), 22–23
ventromedial prefrontal cortex (VMPFC), 16
virtual reality, 102
virtual yoga, 171
VMPFC (ventromedial prefrontal cortex), 16
VMpo (ventral medial nucleus, posterior), 22–23
VNS (vagus nerve stimulation), 97
vocational services, 121

weighting, treatment, 42, 43f
whole health, 169
Whole Health initiative (VA), 169
withdrawal, protracted, 157–58
World Health Organization Composite International Diagnostic Interview, 46–47